S0-BDP-536

ENDORSEMENTS

The combination of personal anecdotes, practical guidance and realistic encouragement Howard Bressler provides in *The Layman's Guide to Surviving Cancer* has resulted in a powerful and inspiring must-read book for any cancer patient and their loved ones navigating through the cancer experience. I highly recommend it.

Joseph I. Lieberman
Former United States Senator and Vice Presidential Candidate

In my forty-five years as a practicing oncologist, I could impart to my patients only a small part of the wisdom expressed in Howard Bressler's outstanding book for cancer patients. He covers everything that is important, and this book should and will become "The Bible" for patients who have been diagnosed with cancer. It will serve as the switch that will turn on the light of understanding, knowledge, pathways of thinking and action, and most importantly, self-fulfillment in the face of a daunting obstacle. My successor oncologists will have one great advantage over me: they will have this vital volume to recommend to patients. I wish I had this book long ago to give to my own patients.

If you are newly diagnosed with cancer, or are already in this new world you did not ask for, read this book from cover to cover. A new world of understanding, positive action, and peace awaits you. This book is truly "Everyone's Guide" to dealing with cancer.

Malin Dollinger, MD, FACP
Clinical Professor of Medicine
Keck School of Medicine, University of Southern California
Author of *Everyone's Guide to Cancer Therapy: How Cancer is Diagnosed, Treated, and Managed Day to Day*

The diagnosis and treatment of cancer, even when the outcome is successful, is often an extraor~~...~~

South Haven Public Library
403 West 700 North
Valparaiso, IN 46385

challenging experience for a patient. The physical, emotional and financial toll on the patient, family and friends is often huge, and there has been no good published guide to help prepare all those involved for what lies ahead.

Howard Bressler has gone a long way toward helping affected people through this daunting period of their lives. He has written an easy-to-read, engaging, commonsense guide for the newly diagnosed cancer patient and those undergoing treatment, based on his own personal battle against leukemia. He combines his own experiences, anecdotes and perspectives to create a practical guide that is positive, proactive and often humorous, and that will inspire and lead other cancer patients through the grueling minefield of the world of cancer. As someone who has spent his career treating cancer patients, I expect to enthusiastically recommend this book to my newly diagnosed patients and those of my colleagues. A terrific read!

Mark Weinblatt, MD
Chief, Division of Pediatric Hematology/Oncology
Director, Cancer Center for Kids
Winthrop University Hospital, Mineola, New York
Professor of Clinical Pediatrics
Stony Brook University School of Medicine

Howard Bressler has accomplished what few have in writing a cancer-related book; he has crafted a work that provides important, practical information, with interesting references, while flowing naturally and being easy to read and understand. Any reader will relate in some form to this book, as Howard describes his emotional and intellectual journey that transforms sorrow and anxiety into hope and life enrichment while he beats leukemia. Furthermore, he presents a step-by-step guide for individuals who receive a shocking cancer diagnosis, and provides invaluable tools that not only will assist them in getting through their treatment but also emerging with a renewed sense of positivity, perspective and purpose. This is a book that every cancer patient should read and it is one that I will recommend with confidence to my own patients and colleagues.

Fernando J. Bianco, MD
Associate Professor of Urology
Department of Urology, Columbia University
Founder, Columbia University Division of Urology at Mount Sinai Medical Center

As an Oncology Nurse who has overseen the treatment of hundreds of cancer patients and has watched them go through the travails of dealing with their disease, I would recommend this book to anyone diagnosed with and being treated for cancer. Howard Bressler has used his personal experiences, struggles, insights and coping strategies, as well as extensive research, to create a practical, easily relatable road map that truly depicts the cancer experience and will direct other cancer patients along their journeys. The stories he tells, the personal thoughts and feelings he relates and the perspectives he has gained as a cancer patient and survivor bring the reader into his world and will open the eyes not only of cancer patients and their families, but of the professionals who treat them. While not hiding from the rigors and realism of the cancer experience, this book still manages to bring a proactive feeling of hope into the equation, and it is one that I believe the patients I work with, as well as my colleagues, will benefit greatly from.

Jennifer Cuevo, RN, MSN, OCN

For many people, a cancer diagnosis is devastating news. I know this from my own experience. So many of us feel terrified and don't know where to turn. So many questions face us as cancer patients: Do I have any control over this extremely traumatic problem? How do I choose the right doctor? What treatment options are best for me? What should I expect? It can be difficult even figuring out where to start.

This book is a terrific guide to help newly diagnosed or current cancer patients deal with the difficulties that all patients will inevitably face during their treatment and on the road back to health. It is both optimistic and honest. No matter what form of cancer a person has, Howard Bressler's insights, suggestions and experiences will relate to them and greatly help them during the treatment process. Additionally, his recommendations as to how to manage one's treatment are essential to anyone who may be unsure of what to do. It's the kind of book I wish I had had when I was first diagnosed with cancer. Bravo!

David Klein
Hodgkin's lymphoma survivor

This book has been an enormous help to me during my treatment and especially during those difficult days in the hospital. It contains so much useful information and advice that I have been able to put into practice in my own battle, and at the same time is so easy to read and relatable. Having been written by someone who has actually "been there" and has gone through his own cancer ordeal, it truly speaks to fellow cancer patients and future survivors.

Gisela Miceli
Ovarian cancer patient

THE LAYMAN'S GUIDE TO SURVIVING CANCER

FROM DIAGNOSIS THROUGH TREATMENT AND BEYOND

THE LAYMAN'S GUIDE TO SURVIVING CANCER

FROM DIAGNOSIS THROUGH TREATMENT AND BEYOND

PORTER COUNTY PUBLIC LIBRARY

South Haven Public Library
403 West 700 North
Valparaiso, IN 46385

HOWARD L. BRESSLER

sabnf   SH
362.19699 BRESS

Bressler, Howard L
The layman's guide to surviving
33410013285251   02/18/15

Copyright © 2014 by Howard Bressler

Langdon Street Press
322 First Avenue N, 5th floor
Minneapolis, MN 55401
612.455.2293
www.langdonstreetpress.com

All rights reserved. No part of this publication may be reproduced, stored in a retrieval system, or transmitted, in any form or by any means, electronic, mechanical, photocopying, recording, or otherwise, without the prior written permission of the author.

MEDICAL DISCLAIMER
The information contained in this book is intended for general information and encouragement only. Individuals should always consult with their doctor or other health-care provider before undertaking, administering or rejecting any treatment, dietary, lifestyle or other suggestions made in this book. Any use or application of the material contained in this book is at the reader's sole discretion and is his or her sole responsibility.

LEGAL DISCLAIMER
Any discussion in this book regarding legal rights or practical recommendations to protect your legal rights are for general informational purposes only and are not to be construed as legal advice. No attorney-client relationship is anticipated or created by any statements in this book and no statements herein are designed to create any such relationship. Readers are encouraged to consult with their own attorneys regarding the protection of their legal rights in connection with their cancer treatment, employment issues or financial or estate planning. Any use or application of the material contained in this book is at the reader's sole discretion and is his or her sole responsibility.

ISBN-13: 978-1-62652-858-1
LCCN: 2014939265

Distributed by Itasca Books

Cover Design by Steve Porter and Howard Bressler
Typeset by James Arneson

Screenplay excerpt from *Men In Black* courtesy of Columbia Pictures

Excerpt from *Alone on a Wide Wide Sea* used with permission

Excerpt from *It's Always Something* by Gilda Radner reprinted with the permission of Simon & Schuster Publishing Group and by permission of ICM Partners, Inc., Copyright © [] by Gilda Radner.

Excerpt from *The Girls' Guide to Hunting and Fishing* by Melissa Bank used with the permission of The Friedrich Agency.

Excerpt from R. Buckman, "Providing Emotional Support" in L. Yount, *Cancer (Contemporary Issues Companion)*, reprinted with permission.

Excerpts reproduced from *Buy Green Bananas*, by Rabbi Berel Wein, with permission of the copyright holders, ArtScroll/Mesorah Publications, Ltd.

Excerpts from M. Dollinger, *Everyone's Guide to Cancer Therapy: How Cancer is Diagnosed, Treated, and Managed Day to Day* (4th U.S. Ed. 2002), used with permission.

Printed in the United States of America

ACKNOWLEDGMENTS

More than anything, this book is an exercise in being thankful: thankful for the chance to experience so much for which there was no foregone conclusion I would have a chance to experience, thankful to have the opportunity to create a vehicle to help others and thankful to those who helped get me here. There are many people to thank for their love, friendship and assistance over the years since my diagnosis and in connection with the writing of this book. While it is my wish to acknowledge specifically all those who have helped me along the way, I apologize in advance to anyone who inadvertently may be overlooked in my gratitude.

- To Dr. Stuart Lichtman, who diagnosed, treated and helped heal me. You approached my care with an open mind and open heart, and that made a huge difference.
- To the wonderful nurses, supervisors and staff at North Shore University Hospital who cared for me on a daily basis and gave me the encouragement that helped get me through each day.
- To the people I never even met who gave me their blood when my own was no good. The short time you gave of yourselves has given me years.
- To my wonderful friends in West Hempstead, who rallied to the aid of my family in its time of great need; who cooked for us, shopped for us, babysat for us and gave us their love. You confirmed the wisdom of our choice in moving to West Hempstead in the first place.

To my colleagues at Kasowitz, Benson, Torres & Friedman, LLP, whose patience and understanding took an enormous weight off my mind and shoulders throughout and since my cancer treatment, and who continue to worry over me like a Jewish grandmother:

- To Marc Kasowitz, who personifies the fact that success and power are not hindered, but rather are enhanced, by compassion. Thank you for giving me a chance and continuing to believe in me.
- To Dan Benson, who taught me the value and power of words, be they professional or personal, how to use them effectively and to write without ego. Your warmth, friendship and red-pen lessons have given me the ability to hopefully help others with my words.
- To Jack Atkin, whose guidance in the practice of law has been so important, but whose guidance in the practice of life has been invaluable. You teach me every day how to be a mensch. I hope some of it has taken hold. And to Rifky Atkin, who knows where I have been and whose perseverance has been a great example to me.
- To Aaron Marks, who may have been one year behind me in graduating from law school, but who far exceeds me in intelligence, achievement and kindness.
- To Andy Davenport, who inspires me to be a better person and reaffirms for me the value of learning from all people.
- To David Shapiro, who gives me the opportunities to reaffirm my perspectives on life.

To my many friends who have stood by me through the years:

- To Rabbi Yehuda Pearl, my teacher and friend, whose insight and honesty have helped this book come to fruition.
- To Jeff Eisenberg, who has mentored me in so many ways, and who taught me the value of charity and how to overcome personal hardships.
- To Seth Greenberg, who has given me more belly laughs than anyone I have ever known. I can always turn to you when I need a good friend and a good laugh. You are the Jake to my Elwood.
- To Mickey Silberman, who always challenges me to think outside the box.

- To Eddie Lowenthal, whose steady friendship over more than two decades has been a great source of strength to me.
- To Sara Goldman, who loves me despite my faults and who always welcomed me into her home during those many days of treatment.
- To Jani Cooperberg, who has a talent for showing up whenever I need her most. It is no coincidence that your maiden name is "Kind."
- To Michael and Miriam Gordon, our first new friends in West Hempstead; your sincerity drew us to you and has kept us close to you since we met.
- To M. D. Laufer, who literally bled for me.
- To Ari Brown, who has helped me realize the value of redemption and reconciliation in the wake of my cancer.
- And to Barry Shuter; your footsteps no longer leave an imprint in the sand, but I still felt you walking beside me throughout the writing of this book. Although I can no longer hear your voice, its echo continues to reverberate.

To my incredible family, for everything, all the time:

- To Mom and Dad, who never outgrew me and whom I have never really outgrown, for all of the lessons, the amazing example you set about serving others and for the many long days and nights in the hospital when I needed you to be there.
- To my sisters, Barbara and Annette. The jokes you have played on your little brother are so far outweighed by the love and support I have received from you over the years. To Barbara, who has shown me how to keep faith during hardships. To Annette, who has shown me the importance of living according to one's ideals.
- To my brothers-in-law, Michael, Josh, Simon and Henry, for treating me like a brother when I never had one.

- To my mother-in-law, for her caring, all of the recipes I tried out during my convalescence and, most of all, for giving me Ceci.
- To Aunt Erma, for showing me that life is better with puppet shows and for always striving for a bigger picture. To Uncle Bob, for always really listening. To my cousins Karen, Cindy and Suzanne, for their guidance in helping to craft this book and for helping me be a good husband by making me "marry" them over and over when we were children.
- To my cousin Ron Esposito. We came from different places, grew together through a shared battle and understood each other as only comrades in arms can. I hope that this book honors your memory.
- To Daniella and Michal. You gave me my biggest reason to live. The worth of everything I had to go through to get here is confirmed every time I see you smile, hear you laugh and get your hugs and kisses. Every milestone I am able to see you through is a victory. Thank you, Michal, for putting your poetic skills to work in assisting me in choosing the quotes for each chapter's introduction.
- And to Ceci, my wife, partner, confidant, best friend and love of my life. Being married to me, with all of its obstacles, has been no easy task, yet you always rise to the occasion. You remain, as you were when I met you all those years ago and through more than two decades of marriage, a woman of infinite charm. I stand in awe of your ability to bring warmth everywhere you go and to touch people in a way no one else can. The journey would not have been worthwhile if you were not traveling it with me. The road ahead is bright because you are walking by my side.

CONTENTS

FOREWORD

I first met Howard Bressler in the summer of 2000. He was referred to me because his general practitioner had run blood tests on him that indicated that his white blood cell and platelet counts were very low. I examined him, ran additional tests and advised him that a bone marrow biopsy was the best way to determine if there was something seriously wrong. I performed the biopsy on him and, later that afternoon, had to do something that every oncologist dreads having to do: I told him that he had cancer, specifically acute promyelocytic leukemia. The next day, he was in the hospital under my care and we began his treatment. It was an arduous course that involved a month-long hospital stay, continued chemotherapy for the better part of a year and a then-experimental treatment protocol which ultimately achieved the desired result for Howard (and others): complete remission.

I have treated hundreds of cancer patients over the years. What stands out to me about Howard and how he dealt with his diagnosis and treatment was his unflagging good spirit, his sense of humor in the face of a difficult diagnosis (often joking his way through additional bone marrow biopsies and greeting me and the nurses who treated him with a consistent smile), his commitment to his family, his genuine faith and daily prayers, his readiness to undertake and follow his treatment regimen and his simple, dogged determination to survive. They all served him well in his cancer battle.

Cancer patients invariably face a number of questions and concerns when they are diagnosed and go through their treatment. Among them are what they will encounter along the way, how their treatments will likely affect them, what they can do to manage the effects of their treatments and how they can manage their affairs and relationships with their loved ones during the course of their battle. What has been missing from the scene is a convenient, straightforward source to help guide them through these issues. Howard Bressler has created that source. In *The Layman's Guide to Surviving Cancer,* he has combined the wisdom and emotion of his personal experience with extensive research to create an informative book that offers useful advice, humor and encouragement to light the way for other patients and their loved ones. His book walks the fine line between personal memoir and practical roadmap unlike any other cancer-related book. I have no doubt that many cancer patients will find the guidance and support they are looking for in these pages. A masterful job.

Stuart M. Lichtman, MD, FACP
Attending Physician
Memorial Sloan-Kettering Cancer Center
Professor of Medicine
Weill Cornell Medical College

PREFACE

It is my hope in writing this book to provide fellow cancer patients and future survivors, as well as their loved ones, with a practical, layman's guide to approaching, treating and surviving their cancer. If you have just been diagnosed with cancer, are undergoing your treatment or you are a supporting family member or friend of a cancer patient, you may be going through the most stressful, uncharted part of your life to date. Take a deep breath. Now, take another. The road, though winding and bumpy, is neither too long nor too arduous for you to travel. And as Lao Tzu said, "A journey of a thousand miles begins with a single step." Each step along that journey, even if it is painful, brings you closer to that destination.

Through my own experiences, those of my family and those of others who have faced their challenges, I have put together what I hope are commonsense, easy-to-apply approaches to dealing with your cancer. I do not intend to suggest that any one course of treatment is better than another. Although throughout this book I discuss various alternative or complementary treatment approaches, there remains significant debate within the medical/scientific community regarding the efficacy of these approaches in preventing, treating or curing cancer. Similarly, while, as I discuss, many people believe—and there is scientific evidence to support the belief—that such things as diet, stress, faith, mood and rest can affect the development, progression and ultimate defeat of cancer, these issues also remain subject to ongoing study and debate. In fact, in addition to the studies I cite, there also are many additional studies (some of which I also cite) that either fail to demonstrate the relevance of these issues to cancer progression and treatment or suggest that improving or controlling these aspects of one's behavior and emotions does not improve the likelihood of surviving cancer.

The treatment approach you use, be it conventional cancer treatment such as chemotherapy, radiation or surgery, alternative medicine or a combination of conventional and alternative approaches—or whether you undergo treatment at all—is something that you will have to decide for yourself. Before you make any decision as to whether to undergo or refrain from any particular treatments, or pursue any alternative approaches to healing, consult your doctor and loved ones to make sure that the choice is best for you. This book also is not meant to be a comprehensive guide to all possible treatments or the nuances of specific types of cancers. Indeed, one of the reasons why cancer causation and treatment are such complex issues is because cancer is not one disease. Rather, there are hundreds of different types of cancers, with varied causes and treatments, a full discussion of which is well beyond the scope of what I can—or want to—do here. There are many other fine, detailed books by other authors more qualified to provide that kind of information, some of which are referred to herein. I received similar books from friends when I was diagnosed, and I was thankful for them, but they were long. They were overly detailed. They were full of complicated statistics. They were denser than my mind was willing to entertain in the throes of my diagnosis. All I really wanted to know was what was going to happen to me and how I could get through it.

In short, what I could have used most when I went through my own cancer and treatment was some of the straightforward advice I try to lay out here. With my own experiences in mind, it was not my intention or desire to write a tome filled with facts, figures and plans. Rather, I have designed this book to be what I wish I had had when I was going through my cancer and what many cancer patients long for: something easy to digest. While I have included many personal anecdotes, this book was not crafted to tell *my* story; it was created to help *you* craft *yours*.

My greatest wish is that it will help alleviate some of your fears and pain, and give you the encouragement to face and defeat whatever demons you may meet along the way.[1]

---

1   At certain points in this book I refer to personal experiences involving specific people. I have changed their names to protect their privacy.

INTRODUCTION

Life was good. Life was *very* good. I had a fascinating, attractive, devoted wife, two beautiful, healthy, young daughters and a nice house. I had a good job and all of the material things I needed. Maybe life was *too* good. Something nagged subconsciously at me. I was named after a great-uncle's son who died when he was twenty-six. He, in turn, had been named after my grandfather's brother, who died when he was seventeen. Lurking somewhere in the recesses of my mind was the idea that I was destined for a short life too. Yet, I had sailed through the first thirty-three years of my life with few hitches. Although my family was far from rich and I grew up in a very middle-class home, my parents worked hard and sacrificed to give me and my sisters whatever we truly needed. I went to private schools, studied abroad for a year, graduated from law school and, for the most part, had an easy upbringing.

As I grew into adulthood, marriage and fatherhood, my only malady was the general feeling of invincibility that many young people—particularly young men—suffer from, with all of the attendant symptoms: excess in too many things and an unhealthy lifestyle. I paid little attention to what I ate or drank. Like many New York lawyers, I thrived on the amount of hours I worked and prided myself on the amount of stress I could endure. I could do these things and live this way because "life was good." Perhaps I had skirted any bad luck connected with the name that had been passed on to me by my two unfortunate ancestors. My faith in God came easily because there was nothing to shake or challenge it. Indeed, life was going so smoothly that I asked my wife, on a few occasions, "When is the other shoe going to drop?" For a while it seemed like it never would. Then it did.

August 23, 2000. Many cancer survivors can remember precisely the date of their diagnosis. That was mine. After feeling run-down, sick and feverish for a couple of weeks, I went to my family doctor and suggested he run a blood test to see if maybe I had an infection. The next day, Saturday, he left me a message on my answering machine telling me that my white blood cell counts were very low; so low, in fact, that if they were any lower he would have had me hospitalized. In all likelihood there was something viral going on, so I gave it another week. When I did not improve, I had another full workup done, with the same results. Finally, my mother referred me to a hematological oncologist at North Shore University Hospital on Long Island, who had treated my grandmother. He ran a blood test and told me that, although my white blood cell count had remained essentially the same from the previous tests (too low), my platelets had fallen off about 50 percent over the previous week. He told me that we could wait and retest in a few days to see if there was any improvement or I could have a bone marrow biopsy to see what was going on.

I was not interested in waiting anymore. Had I known what a bone marrow biopsy feels like (particularly when you are sick) I might have thought otherwise, but we went ahead with the test. To this day, it was the single most painful physical experience I have had. For those of you who have never enjoyed one, imagine someone twisting a corkscrew into your hip bone and then sucking out your marrow. Still, the doctor said on initial review that my cell structure looked good, and I felt relatively confident that I would be okay. Later that afternoon, however, he called and spoke the following words: "I'm afraid the news is not good." Now, when your regular doctor calls you and says something is not good, it could be anything: a bounced check; the insurance denied your request for plastic surgery;

you're really a woman. But when your oncologist calls you with that kind of news, things are bad.

Immediately, I was on my feet and pacing around my room while my wife watched and listened nervously. *Leukemia.* Acute promyelocytic leukemia (or APL for short). In an instant, everything I had come to expect was thrown into disarray. Everything that I thought was settled—my family life, my relationships, my job, my very meaning and place in this world—became suddenly unhinged. As if I was experiencing my own, personal earthquake, the ground under me unexpectedly had opened into a chasm and I felt myself thrust onto the ledge of a cliff that had risen up out of nowhere. *Cancer. Me.* My God, what did it mean? Was this the early end whose prospect had nagged at some part of me for years? Was I going to die? Would I live long enough to see my daughters grow up? Would I live long enough for them even to be able to *remember* me?

It was like a tornado in my head for a few moments; a "deer in the headlights" experience. When my head cleared I asked my doctor simply, "Where do we go from here?" He told me that I would be going into the hospital the next day, that I would be there for at least a month, and that I would have to undergo chemotherapy. It was, needless to say, a lot to absorb. But, he said, "Although I don't want to minimize the seriousness of your disease, the cure rate is high."

So I went to the hospital and, as he predicted, I spent a month there. I went through treatment over the course of the next year. I took part in a protocol that treated my APL with an established chemotherapy regimen and arsenic trioxide, which was then an experimental treatment. I lost my hair. I was sicker than I ever thought I could be. I had many moments of doubt and fear but far more moments of hope and faith. I had my family and friends to support me. I had my belief in God to sustain me. I had great nurses and a doctor who cared. I had colleagues and bosses who supported me and reassured me that I could take all of the time I needed to get well without pressure to return to work before I was ready to do so. I had my wife and daughters to live for. So I lived. I survived.

Many people have asked me why I waited more than a decade since my treatment ended to write this book. The truth is that, like many cancer survivors, the initial thrill of survivorship had me thinking about writing an inspiring, humorous, enlightening book about my experiences. But life retook me and those good intentions slipped into the wake of living again. My reactions to being "cured" were not entirely uncommon, albeit not the healthiest. Like many cancer survivors, what I felt more than anything was a sense of entitlement. I had lived. I had endured a month of hospitalization and months of chemotherapy. I had dealt with the uncertainty of my future. Now I deserved everything. So I indulged. I ate what I wanted to eat (all of the things I could neither taste nor stomach during the throes of chemotherapy). I drank what I wanted to drink. I smoked expensive cigars. I bought the sports car I had always wanted.

But those things were counterproductive (except the sports car—no regrets there). The wiser choice would have been to take the blessing life had given me (yes, cancer, properly viewed, can be a blessing) and commit myself to treating my body and soul with respect. That is a realization that has come to me in more recent years, as my leukemia has receded into further—albeit ever-present—memory. Another curse-turned-potential-blessing has been my subsequent battle with Stevens-Johnson Syndrome, which has given me the greater impetus to focus not only on being healthy but acting to preserve that health. That battle led me to pursue a healthier lifestyle, both in terms of my physical health and my spiritual path, and led me to begin work on this book.

For the past two decades I have worked as a lawyer, with a heavy emphasis on "toxic tort" cases; in other words, cases that involve people who claim that their injuries—including, in many cases, various types of cancer—were caused by their exposure to chemicals and other toxic substances. Much of what I have done over the years involved analyzing whether those people's injuries could be linked scientifically and medically to their claimed exposures. I spent a lot of my time researching what causes various diseases, debunking theories that could not stand up to the science or the evidence and working with medical and other scientific experts to better understand what had caused, or did not cause, the disease in question. Indeed, one of the things that I liked best about my job was that it kept me on the cutting edge and forced me to learn new areas of science with each case. As such, by the time I was diagnosed with leukemia—and, even more so, in the ensuing decade—I had honed the skills to delve into the science behind disease and gain an enhanced understanding of how the body acts in encountering and fighting a disease-causing agent.

When I was first diagnosed, I put those skills to work in investigating and pursuing answers as to the possible effects of my treatment. I looked at studies analyzing the causes and effects of APL. I researched and asked pointed questions about the side effects of the drugs that I was to take. The intervening years since I finished my treatments have been filled with additional professional focus on both pursuing and defending against personal injury, toxic tort claims, including more cancer claims, learning, with each case, more about not only the science of those claims but also the human, emotional and psychological components involved in battling disease. In helping people prepare their cases for trial, I have had to take them through their own cancer journeys and help them tell their stories. I have seen how they, like I, continue to feel and deal with the full emotions of cancer, even years after they have completed their treatments, and how cancer changed their lives. In fact, my perspectives on such claims have taken on a much broader and more personal dimension since my own cancer battle. That additional experience, viewed through the lens of my own cancer ordeal, has proved vital to gaining an understanding of the various mechanisms of disease and possible routes to healing—medical, emotional and spiritual—laid out in this book. Indeed, I believe that, viewed through the prism of the last ten years of reflection and continued battles, as well as my continued work in addressing the claims of people I have encountered in my legal practice, this book is a more mature work than it would have been had I written it earlier in my career or in the surreal haze of a recent cancer ordeal.

It is my hope that my experiences and the words in this book will make your cancer, or the cancer of your loved one, easier; that it will help you sooner embark on the path to health and rebirth, as you prepare for the rest of your life. It is of foremost importance that you remember, and always keep in mind, that, as Dr. Robert Buckman wrote, "Cancer is a word. It's not a sentence."[2] It may be a dirty word, but it is one that can be cleansed.

---

2   R. Buckman, *Cancer is a Word, Not a Sentence*, 11.

PART I

GET READY TO RUMBLE

Dealing With Your Diagnosis and Going Through Treatment

CHAPTER 1

FIRST THINGS FIRST:
YOU'VE BEEN DIAGNOSED, NOW WHAT?

*"There are some words that my mother finds too
horrible to utter, so she whispers them."*

Mare Winningham to Rob Lowe in *St. Elmo's Fire*

Being told that you have cancer can be a devastating piece of news. This is because, rightly or wrongly, many of us have come to understand cancer as a death sentence. So frightening is a cancer diagnosis that the disease is often talked about only in hushed whispers. Indeed, I can recall a scene from the movie *St. Elmo's Fire* where Mare Winningham's character pulls Rob Lowe aside before a family dinner and tells him that "there are some words that my mother finds too horrible to utter, so she whispers them." And, sure enough, the mother says, "Did you hear about Billy Rothberg? [In a harsh whisper] *Cancer.*" So foul and blasphemous a word is cancer that it is afforded the same treatment as some of the most obscene words in our vernacular. Just as the most offensive racial epithet is referred to as the "N-word," and the most foul obscenity is called the "F-word," cancer is often shunned as the "C-word," never to be uttered in full, lest we be tainted by it.

But cancer is not an obscenity. It is not contagious. It is not stigmatizing. It need not be muttered only in undertones and in the fear that someone else might hear us say it. That is because cancer is not necessarily a death sentence. It is indeed an enemy; one that needs to be attacked and routed. But it is not an insurmountable one by any stretch of the imagination. How we absorb the news of a cancer diagnosis, plot our defense (and, moreover, our *offense*) against it, live with it, help our loved ones and friends live with it and, ultimately, defeat it, will demonstrate that this is so.

I can recall quite clearly the whirlwind in my head when my oncologist told me my diagnosis. I know he told me exactly the type of leukemia that I had but I was at a loss to repeat it accurately. I felt dizzy, woozy and scared. My heart started beating hard and my stomach knotted up. In my life and my career as a lawyer, I had always thrived in situations in which I had a grip on all of the facts; where things were usually rational and I could often control or at least have a say in controlling developments. But this diagnosis seemed to be in diametric opposition to all of that. I did *not* grasp all of the facts. I felt initially that I was *not* in control. It was all simply irrational, and I was not prepared. Almost immediately, I began to pace the room as if perhaps I could shake off the stain with which I had just been painted. And I can recall the anguished look on my wife's face and her pitifully sad, "I knew it!"

But when that initial rush of vertigo passed (and it passed rather quickly), everything seemed clear to me—the danger, the challenges, the hope for survival and the reality that I might not survive. All of these things crystallized very quickly in my mind, and I can recall how calmly I asked my doctor how we needed to proceed. Whatever I had to do, I would do it. In a split second I had cleared my brain and seen that my path to health lay before me, if I had the courage to take it on without quarter and fight my cancer continuously and without end until *it* was dead and *I* was alive.

And that is the first thing you must do; clear your thinking so that you can make your plans. You will need to take steps to reduce your stress and fear. That may not be so easy to do. Our bodies are designed to react in a particular manner to danger, and being told you have cancer can trigger that reaction. Your body may undergo a stress response, generating a burst of adrenaline. You may feel a rush of anger or be frozen into immediate inaction or inability to react, just as you might react if you were threatened by a dangerous animal or a criminal attack.

In fact, when a person is under stress, essential body functions that may be necessary to combat cancer—including the immune and digestive systems—largely switch off, so that all of the body's energies can be directed toward the stressing stimulus.[3] Indeed, the effect of stress—particularly the stress that flows from aggressive feelings or confrontations—is to stimulate an inflammatory physiological response that some people believe, and some studies suggest, may even enhance the growth of cancerous tumors.[4] The ability of our natural killer cells to combat diseases is blocked by the hormones (such as cortisol and noradrenaline) released when we feel stressed.[5] Thinking clearly and calmly is very difficult when you are in this condition. You may experience a period, be it hours or even days, when you feel incapable of making any

---

3   See R. Gorter and E. Peper, *Fighting Cancer: A Nontoxic Approach to Treatment*, 25.

4   D. Servan-Schreiber, MD, PhD, *Anticancer: A New Way of Life*, 141. *See also* S. Reuter, et al., "Oxidative Stress, Inflammation and Cancer: How are they Linked?" *Free Radoc. Biol. Med.* (December 1, 2010): 49(11): 1603–1616 (stating that "oxidative stress, chronic inflammation, and cancer are closely linked"); R. Skopec, "Mechanism Linking Aggression Stress through Inflammation to Cancer," *J. Cancer Sci Ther* (2011): 3:6: 134–139 at pp. 134–135, 137.

5   *Anticancer*,142.

decisions regarding your treatment, or perhaps you will feel like you do not even want to deal with it at all. These reactions are all normal.

The fact remains, however, that you need to get past that initial reaction. As Vince Lombardi, the famous Green Bay Packers football coach, once said, "It's not whether you get knocked down, it's whether you get up." You need to see clearly what your fight is and begin to clarify in your mind and with the help of your doctors and others the path you must take to win. It is likely that the road you see will, like my own, be uneven and strewn with obstacles that might seem from far away to be immovable and insurmountable. They are not. You will find that when you get up close, nose to nose with them, and then inevitably climb past them, they were never quite the impenetrable barriers you thought they were.

Getting your bodily and emotional systems back online is a prerequisite to undertaking your treatment and fighting your cancer effectively. There are many ways to do so, and you will need to pick one or several that work for you.

Breathe

When you are feeling overwhelmed, stepping back and spending several minutes doing some deep, purposeful breathing, in a quiet environment, can often help you cleanse your mind. It slows your heart rate and forces more oxygen into your body and mind. It can help you focus. Find a peaceful place where you will not be bothered and try this technique: Focus on things that are pleasant and the reasons you have to overcome your cancer, whether it is enjoying your children, reaching milestones with your family or doing things you've always wanted to do.

A good technique to incorporate into your breathing is to purposefully tense the various muscle groups in your body and focus on releasing specific muscle areas as you exhale slowly. Clench and then feel your fists unclenching. Lift and then feel your shoulders droop in relaxation. Feel the tension in your face being released and your brow releasing its furrows. Practice breathing in measured intervals: for example by breathing in through your nose deeply for five seconds, holding for three seconds, releasing for five seconds and then waiting three more seconds before taking the next breath. This process will slow your heartbeat and calm you down. Slow yourself down, and your mind will start to clear.

Move

Physical exercise causes the body to release endorphins (which in turn improve our mood) and reduces stress. It helps us release pent-up energy that comes from the body's stress response to stimuli that worry or frighten us, and will help dissipate some of the adrenal response you are experiencing. Even gentle exercise can do these things.

If you are still physically strong and have a workout routine, do it. If you are feeling weak, which may be the case if you have been diagnosed with cancer, do some very gentle exercises. Walking is particularly good, especially in a relaxing environment. If you live near a park or beach, those are excellent choices not only for relieving your physical stress and easing your mind, but gathering your thoughts without the distractions that can come from busier environments. If someone is available to whom you feel particularly close or whose opinion you value, ask that person to go with you and share his thoughts with you.

If you cannot get outside, do some gentle stretching routines, regulating your breathing as you do so. This too can remarkably lessen stress. Even if you cannot get out of bed, there are exercises you can do to help you de-stress. Sitting in a comfortable position, use the tension-release method described above. Focus on flexing the various muscle areas in your body, including your arms, legs, back and shoulders, and then feel yourself consciously releasing and relaxing each area, all while breathing deeply and slowly. Doing this exercise several times not only relaxes you but also works your muscles.

Accept

If you are going through a sense of denial or are having trouble accepting that this could happen to you, you need to accept your cancer. Some of what you are feeling may be due to guilt. It is common for cancer patients to feel that they have "done something" to bring on their disease. This may include physical actions or omissions (e.g., smoking, overeating, failing to exercise) or perceived spiritual failings (that you are being "punished" for something you did wrong).

Bear in mind that there are many aspects involved in getting cancer, including your heredity and environment, over which you have absolutely no control. And if you have lived a lifestyle that has contributed to your cancer, *forgive yourself.* If you would forgive another person who has wronged you somehow (and most of us can do so), you owe yourself no less consideration. If you helped break it, you can help fix it. You can learn from your mistakes and correct them. Give yourself permission to be scared, to cry and to shout a bit. Accept your situation. Once you have done so, you will find that the emotional path to tackling your treatment will become clearer.

Counsel

The people you love and trust will be there for you. The time we invest in those we love realizes the greatest return when we are in trouble. Trust them. Tell them how you are feeling, whether it is angry, depressed or frightened. There will be many times down the road when you will break down and they will see the nakedness of your fear, and there is no shame in that.

When I received my own diagnosis, the thing that gripped me in fear and longing for someone to turn to was the reality that I would have to leave my children and would not see them again for weeks (if I even got well enough to *ever* see them). Thankfully, the one person I could always turn to and share my feelings with, my wife, Ceci, was next to me, and she sat with me and held me as I unloaded the misery that I was feeling about that issue. Having her there and sharing my emotions with her confirmed what I really already knew: that my partner in life would be my partner in my battle. It made me feel better, even if it did not wholly alleviate my concerns. Sharing our feelings gives us a sense of relief; a sense of not being alone in our struggles. It will allow you to feel "unloaded" of the burden of carrying your cancer on your own. As Dr. Buckman wrote in encouraging loved ones to talk to a cancer patient:

> One of the arguments friends and family put forward in order to avoid talking to the patient is that talking about a fear or an anxiety might create that anxiety, even if it didn't exist before the conversation. In other words, a friend might say to herself: "*If I ask my friend whether he's worried about radiotherapy, and he wasn't worried about it, I might make him worried about it.*" Well, that doesn't happen. There is very good evidence from studies done by psychiatrists talking to patients with terminal illnesses ... that conversations between the patients and their relatives and friends did not create new fears or anxieties. In fact, the opposite was true; *not* talking about a fear makes it bigger. Those patients who have nobody to talk to have a higher incidence of anxiety and depression.[6]

---

6   R. Buckman, "Providing Emotional Support," in L. Yount, *Cancer: Contemporary Issues Companion*, 104.

Talk to the Professionals

If you have a spiritual advisor or clergyman with whom you are particularly close, talk to him. They are professionals whose job description involves helping people through difficult, even devastating, life events. Most of us have never used the services of a professional counselor, such as a psychologist, social worker or psychiatrist. Now may be the time to seek professional counseling, and your doctor or hospital administrators may be able to recommend someone experienced in dealing with people who have cancer and are undergoing the emotions often associated with a cancer diagnosis and treatment. There is no shame in seeking out the assistance of such professionals. Indeed, if there was ever a time when such counseling is understandable, it is when you are in the throes of cancer treatment. Young cancer patients may relate better to a teacher or school counselor. If your child has cancer and is close to a certain teacher or principal, enlist that person to help out. Let her reach out gently to your child and give her the avenue for venting her concerns or fears. Ultimately, the only important issue is whether it makes *you*, the patient, feel better. If it does, do it.

Of course, your doctor, be it your general practitioner or oncologist, can provide an invaluable counseling resource. As professionals who spend countless hours studying, diagnosing and treating cancer—as well as witnessing firsthand the difficulties and emotions experienced by cancer patients and their families and, literally and figuratively, holding their hands through treatment—they have a wellspring of experience and knowledge upon which you can draw. If you are fortunate enough to have a doctor with a good "bedside manner," he or she will know how to listen to your concerns, provide you with the information and encouragement you seek and allay your fears. They know what is "normal" in the context of your treatment, what you will likely experience and, often, how you can best get through your trying times. As you go through your treatment, your doctor will probably be best able to prepare you for "what comes next" in terms of side effects or what is going to happen to your body. Indeed, there were numerous times during my own treatment—including when I was at my sickest and most feverish points and when my blood counts dipped frighteningly—when being reassured by my doctor that what I was experiencing was "normal," and that he saw it regularly with similarly situated patients, went further than anything else in making me believe that I would get through it and get well.

Comrades in Arms

You may also feel that someone who has not "been there" cannot really understand your emotions. This is true to some extent, because although our loved ones and friends— and even our oncologists—can sympathize with our cancer battle, only fellow cancer survivors can truly *empathize*. For this reason, you may want to reach out to another survivor to express how you are feeling and gain the benefit of his wisdom, experience and empathy. If you do not know anyone who has had the specific cancer you have or has gone through the specific treatment you are undergoing, ask your doctor or hospital to refer you to someone who has. Speaking with someone who has been where you are— and has emerged out the other side—can be enormously beneficial. Many cancer survivors are more than willing to help others in a similar position. There are also support groups for almost all types of cancer, which can be located either through an Internet search or by consultation with your doctors.

Setting the Mood

In addition, make sure you set the right mood for your counseling. Turn off your cell phone or computer. Take the house phone off the hook. Make sure the television or radio is off. Ask whomever you are speaking with to do the same. Although modern life has afforded us the many conveniences these devices provide, they can be a terrible distraction. When you truly need to counsel with someone, you want to avoid these distractions.

Also, make sure that the person you want to talk to is ready to speak to *you*. Although you may feel a tremendous need to unload to a particular person—especially if it's a family member or loved one—that person may herself feel distressed or depressed about your situation and may simply not be ready to listen as you need her to. She may feel like she just does not know what to say or may be afraid of saying the "wrong thing." She may be emotionally unprepared to see you cry. Ask her plainly, "Can I talk to you?" "Are you ready to listen to how I am feeling?" Ask her to be honest. Speaking about your feelings to someone who has a negative response, either by expressing their own despair or pulling away from you, can make you feel worse, so you may want to delay speaking with that person if she is unable to give you what you need.

Further, tell the person to whom you want to speak what it is you want from her. Do you want to know her advice about how to treat your cancer? Are you going to ask her for favors while you are undergoing treatment? Do you simply want her to listen to you express your fears and frustrations so you can unload your emotions? Do you need a hug? Letting someone know exactly what you need from her makes it easier for her to prepare herself mentally to offer you what you need. It also gives that person a sense of importance in being involved somehow in your recuperation, which loved ones so often need. Sometimes the most helpful thing she can do is simply to be there for you and listen to your fears, anxieties and hopes. Tell her she is helping you by doing so. It will make you and her feel better.

If you are having trouble speaking about what you are feeling or feel a strong need to talk, but simply don't know where to start, tell her. It is all right to say "I am not sure how to start," or "I have so much that I want to say but I just don't know how." It is fine for you to admit to her that "I am not comfortable talking about my feelings," or to say that "I am not the sort of person who normally shares intimate details of my emotions." That in itself will help her feel empowered by the fact that you are choosing to share with *her*, and will begin to free *you* of your hesitancy in opening up.

Lead

As hard as it may be, since you control what treatment you will undergo, you are the leader in your battle against cancer. You are essentially the commanding officer. That may be daunting, but recognizing and embracing that role can also be particularly empowering. Take charge. Call the shots. Just as the morale for an entire company of soldiers about to embark on a dangerous battle will be set by the attitude of its commanding officer, those around you, your friends and loved ones, will gauge the approaching battle through *your* demeanor. If you communicate to them that you are concerned but *confident*, they will be too. You are the leader, and how others follow depends on how well you lead.

Indeed, that kind of proactivity can have a profound effect on your mood and, moreover, the mood of those around you and their ability to help you. As Dr. Gorter noted: "[A] sense of powerlessness can actually suppress your immune system. Research has shown that this can lower your defenses, which allows cancer cells to grow more rapidly."[7] As such, staying proactive and fostering the knowledge that you have within yourself the power to defeat your cancer—that you are far from powerless—is a crucial means of doing so. As Georg Groddeck wrote back in 1923: "One must not forget that recovery is brought about not by the physician, but by the sick man himself. He heals himself, by his own power, exactly as he walks by means of his own power, or eats, or thinks, breathes or sleeps."[8]

A personal anecdote is a case in point. When I went into the hospital, my wife asked if I wanted her to stay with me over the Sabbath. My parents also were planning on coming. "No," I told her, "I want you to maintain as much normalcy for the girls [then only three and a half and one] as possible. Stay home and come to see me Saturday night." It wasn't that I didn't want her there to comfort me; I did. But I took control. I prioritized the reactions of my children, who may or may not have been able to comprehend the enormity of what was going on for them—that Daddy was stuck in a building where he had to take drugs that made him sick—and I sacrificed what I truly wanted for what I wanted *for them*. What I wanted for others—the right priorities and attitudes—I undertook to create myself.

In addition, when offered the choice of pursuing only the conventional treatments for APL or becoming part of an experimental treatment as well, I made the decision to be as aggressive as my body could stand. I took the lead, set the course of action and took control as much as possible over my cancer. Doing so empowered me to take the actions necessary to heal, and showing others that I felt that *I* had control over my situation helped them believe that *they* were in control of their situation with me.

---

7   Gorter, *Fighting Cancer*, 29.
8   G. Groddeck, The Book of the It, Letter 32 (1923).

Put simply, you must endeavor to let the initial shock and fear of a cancer diagnosis wash over and past you as quickly as possible. Stand up, even if it's hard. Push forward, even if it hurts. Be brave, even if, like the rest of us, you're more scared than you have ever been. As the incomparable Mark Twain expressed it best: *"Courage is resistance to fear, mastery of fear—not absence of fear."*

CHAPTER 2

NEXT STEPS

"Take the first step in faith. You don't have to see the whole staircase, just take the first step."
Martin Luther King, Jr.

Once the reality of your cancer has been absorbed as much as possible, there are a myriad of other issues that need to be addressed. Among these are telling the people you love about your diagnosis, preparing yourself mentally and emotionally for the fight of your life and choosing the right doctor to help you do so.

Breaking the News without Breaking Hearts

In today's society, adults are used to hearing bad news. Indeed, bad news from the world, including tragedies of immeasurable proportions, is so commonplace that we often merely shrug off all but the most traumatic events, or experience transient feelings of dismay and sympathy, only to be distracted again when life retakes us. But make no mistake, being somewhat desensitized to bad news does not insulate our loved ones, even grown men and women, from the violent emotions of fear, anger, anxiety and depression that accompany the news that someone they love has cancer, so how we break the news to them is important. In general, though, people are tougher than we often think, and this is all the more so when someone close to them is threatened in some way. How often do we hear of ordinary people accomplishing extraordinary feats when someone they love is in trouble? Mothers lift cars off their children at accident scenes; fathers fight off thugs threatening physical violence; children calmly call 911 when a parent is injured or sick. People often rise to the occasion, and you need not sell your loved ones short in debating when and how to tell them you have cancer.

As is often the case, honesty is usually the best policy. But your honesty should be *informed* honesty. Before hitting your loved ones with "the news," get all of the *reliable* information you can about your specific type of cancer and a good explanation from your doctor as to what you will be going through (your course of treatment, whether you will have to be hospitalized, what the likely prognosis is), as well as a reasonable approximation of what you may need from them. Being ready with this kind of information will avoid a situation where the only information they get from you, in isolation, is the fact that you have cancer. Their getting more information on which to focus and concentrate their energies—both physical and emotional—may lessen the impact of hearing that you have cancer. It will give them the means to be active and involved directly in your decisions and healing process, which will likely be the thing they most want to do.

Of course, breaking the news to people particularly close to you will still be difficult. If you feel the need, ask your doctor to be involved in the conversation. That may help you avoid having to explain some of the more technical details of your disease and treatment and add the perspective of someone who has seen and treated many other cancer patients (and can reassure your loved ones that many survive and go on to lead full lives). If you have a clergyman or spiritual advisor, he too can be involved and help lessen the blow. Such advisors generally have a lot more experience than most laypeople in helping others work their way through hardships and grief. The bottom line is, if you doubt your ability to tell your loved ones by yourself that you have cancer, you do not have to *be* alone. You are about to start a road on which you will likely need help from others, and there is no shame in asking for that help immediately.

That having been said, how should you break the news? First, unless someone who needs to be told is far away, have your discussion face-to-face. Hearing that you have cancer will unnerve your loved ones just as it unnerved you. It is best, therefore, and safest, to wait until a spouse comes home from work or a child comes home from school. It may be difficult in today's instantaneous world to resist calling someone on a cell phone or texting them, especially when you feel, justifiably, the need to share what's happened and have the support of those you trust most. But rattling the world of someone who has to then drive home, or causing him to hear devastating news (and the inevitable emotional trauma that ensues) at work or school does him no good. Moreover, the first thing he will likely want to do is embrace you, and hearing the news at a distance will only frustrate him and you, as you will be deprived of that affection when you need it most. So, although it is hard, wait until the soonest "right time" to tell the people you love what is going on.

Telling your parents also can be especially difficult. There is nothing that parents fear as much as the thought of their child being in danger. The call to my parents was troubling, as they were adults (and therefore more able than my children to understand the potential ramifications of my diagnosis), were a couple of hours away from home and were, after all, my parents. I could only imagine what I would feel if, God forbid, one of my children were to bring me such news. I was up front with them but immediately conveyed to them what my doctor had told me about the treatability of my particular form of leukemia, and that seemed to calm them a bit. They promised me they would come home the next day. When I hung up the phone I turned to my wife and said, "They'll be home tonight." Sure enough, they were at my house later that evening, having driven the couple of hours back home.

I only had to tell a few friends, who all received the news with strong words of encouragement and offers to help with whatever they could. The rest of my friends I did not need to tell, because word spread quickly through the community grapevine and, within a couple of hours, one of my oldest friends, who lives in my neighborhood, was at my door, imploring me not to "go through this alone." "Go through it alone?" I asked. "I just found out about it myself." But as with many tough times in life, you will find out when you are diagnosed with and then treated for cancer who your true friends are. If you are not already amazed by the generosity of people, you will be. Do not be afraid or bashful about taking people up on their offers to help, babysit, cook, shop or visit. If you would do it for them (and you would), then you have earned the right to accept help from your friends and loved ones. Indeed, it is a good idea to create a list of things you will likely need help with during your treatment and convalescence so that when people ask what they can do you can assign them a specific task.

Telling the Children

For me, the most difficult conversation was the one I had to have with my children. Getting children to understand that you have cancer and what that means can be very challenging. If they are young, as mine were, they simply may not understand (but *you* will understand the magnitude of what your cancer means for *them*). The conversation I had with my elder daughter, who was all of three and a half at the time, was, in fact, very good and straightforward. She seemed to grasp—at her own level—many of the elements of what was going to be going on with me that I would have thought she could not understand. Our discussion was frank and honest and, for me, the absolute low point of my day before I was to go into the hospital. I explained to her that Daddy was sick and would have to go away the next day to get some treatments in a hospital and that I probably would not be able to see her and her sister for a while. I told her I would probably look different when I came home, that I might lose my hair and lose weight, but that that was just part of getting better. By being honest with her, letting her know gently what was going on and prioritizing the maintenance of her sense of normalcy, I was able to get through it. In general, such honesty encourages a child to ask questions and feel more at ease with a parent's cancer.[9]

Be Reassuring, Be Honest

Children can be affected very significantly by their parent's cancer diagnosis. To a young child, a parent represents everything: strength, consistency, reliability, comfort and courage. She looks up to her parents and sees them on some level as invincible and all-powerful. To hear that her parent is very sick and may have to go to a hospital can be devastating to her, as it can shake her very notion of what can be relied upon in life.

Also, what little your child probably knows about illness is what he or she learns from the colds or strep throat to which they may be exposed by their friends in school. As such, her notion about illness is that she can "catch it" from someone else. As a result, she may develop a fear that your

---

9 See G. H. Christ and A. Christ, "Current Approaches to Helping Children Cope with a Parent's Terminal Illness," *CA: Cancer Guide for Clinicians*, vol. 56, no. 4 (July/August 2006): 197–212. It is available at http://onlinelibrary.wiley.com/doi/10.3322/canjclin.56.4.197/full.

cancer is contagious and either she or your spouse—her other pillar of support—may become infected by it. Reassure her that cancer is not "contagious"; that she cannot catch it from someone who has it. Moreover, most cancers, especially those experienced in childhood, are not inherited genetically. In other words, you should tell your children that just because a parent or sibling has cancer does not mean that *she* will get it.

Your children may also develop anxiety about whether you will die. You need to reassure them that you and the doctors are really attacking your cancer and are doing everything to get rid of it. If you are religious, tell them that many people are praying for you and that is helping. You can even tell them that the physical side effects they may see (vomiting, hair loss or weight loss, for example), show how strong the medicine that you are taking to defeat your cancer is. Preparing them for the physical changes you will undergo will help lessen the shock of your cancer on them.

Telling your children that you definitely will *not* die, however, can have devastating effects on them if you do. Their whole notion of being able to trust their parents or other adult loved ones may be shaken if your promise that you will not die from your cancer is not fulfilled. A better approach to this question may be the one I employed both for myself and others, and which I discuss elsewhere: "I am not going to die today." That will give your child the assurance that you will be there today and tomorrow, and may be enough to allay their fears.

Keep a Finger on Their Emotional Pulse

Children whose parents or siblings are diagnosed with and treated for cancer also may manifest their anxieties in other ways. They may:

- start to have nightmares;
- resume bedwetting;

- want to sleep in your or your spouse's bed;
- become more "clingy" or cry more easily when you or your spouse leaves to go somewhere or when they have to go to school;
- start acting out either in school or at home and start to misbehave or get into fights;
- start to perform poorly in school; or
- even become jealous of the amount of attention bestowed on a sibling with cancer and resent that sibling.

Be very sensitive to these or other changes in your child's behavior or mood. Let his teachers, principals, school counselors and the parents of his friends know what you are going through and ask them to keep an eye open for any change of behavior or mood in your child. You may simply be too distracted to pick up on all of these things, or may not even be home to see them.

Just as you may need to counsel with others or with a professional, your child may need to do so as well. Her school or pediatrician, or your doctor or hospital, should be able to recommend a child psychologist or counselor who can help her. Tell your child also that there are things that she can do to help you feel better, whether that is sending you notes or pictures that you can display in your hospital room, praying for you or doing small jobs around the house. When she comes to visit you in the hospital, have her bring activities to do with you, such as board or video games or reading a favorite book, that she does with you at home. When I went into the hospital, I brought with me some of the Dr. Seuss books that I regularly read with my children so I could read to them over the phone when my immune system was too weak to allow them to visit me. If you are taking oral medication, allow your child to bring it to you and dispense it by giving you the specific pills you need. Getting your child involved in your recovery—and giving her the sense that she is playing an important role in helping you get better—can help alleviate some of the helplessness she may be feeling and resolve some of her anxieties.

Be conscious of the fact that even very young children can be traumatized by your illness, but may be unable to express how they are feeling. Even though my own children were very young when I was diagnosed and went through my chemotherapy, in subsequent years, when I experienced other illnesses, whether routine (like a cold) or more complex (like my episodes of Stevens-Johnson Syndrome), they clearly became anxious over whether my cancer had come back. They expressed their fear that I would have to go back to "the big building" (the hospital).

It is particularly important with such young children to make sure that a substitute caregiver is available with whom they have a strong connection of love and trust.[10] It is vital that, as much as possible, their routine—their sense of normalcy—is not upset. Resist the urge to let them miss school or extracurricular activities. Arrange their regular play dates. Avoid doing things with them that are out of the ordinary or giving in to excess. If your child is not allowed to eat sweets, for example, do not suddenly start indulging him. If he has a regular bedtime, stick to it. Do not let him get too far out of his routine. What you see as kindness or doting in a difficult time itself may alert them to the fact that "something" is wrong. While a child whose parent has cancer may need more attention and affection—and should get it—you should avoid sending the message that something is not right in his world.

In fact, one of the best indicators my wife and I received that this approach was the right one was a comment one of

---

10   Christ and Christ, "Helping Children Cope," 197–212.

my elder daughter's teachers made during my illness: that she could not tell from my daughter's behavior or mood that anything was wrong at home.

Find Your "Why"

Of course, in addition to dealing with the emotions of others, you will have to deal with your own emotions, and the range of those emotions can run the gamut from fear, anxiety, anger and depression. One question that predominates for many cancer patients is "Why me?" This is particularly true where a person has led a healthy lifestyle and has avoided many of the things that lead to cancer, including a sedentary lifestyle or obvious carcinogens, like cigarette smoking. Or someone may feel that they have lived a "good life" and that they "just don't deserve" to be afflicted with cancer. To such people, cancer seems simply "unfair."

Although I also struggled fleetingly with "Why me?" I came to realize that a more appropriate question was, "Why *not* me?" I had to be honest with myself. I recognized that, for me, on a spiritual level, "Why me?" was an audacious question. Indeed, even if I had lived an overall "good life," if there is one thing that historically has been shown, it is that even the most righteous and pious people—people far better than I—sometimes are afflicted or persecuted.

If you are a religious person or study the Bible, you need only look at the biblical patriarchs. Abraham was told to leave his ancestral home and family and go to a strange land hundreds of miles away. He forsook all other gods for the belief in one true God. Finally gifted with children in his old age, he was then instructed to (abortively) sacrifice one son, Isaac, and cast out the other, Ishmael. He also was told that, although his descendants would one day become a "great nation," they first would have to endure hundreds of years of slavery in Egypt. The biblical father of monotheism was given tests that must have taxed his soul greatly.

His son Isaac endured the enmity of his own sons, Jacob and Esau, to each other, was hoodwinked by Jacob (with the complicity of Isaac's wife, Rebecca) into granting him the firstborn blessing, and then had to endure the absence of Jacob for decades and the apostasy of Esau. Jacob, the father of the tribes of Israel, was deceived by his uncle/father-in-law into marrying a woman he did not love (Leah), had to work for fourteen years to marry the woman he *did* love (Rachel) only to see her die in childbirth and endured the seeming loss of his favorite son, Joseph, when Joseph's brothers *sold him into slavery.*

And what of Moses, a man so great that he was charged with receiving the law from God and is the only person that the Bible describes as having spoken with God "face to face?" He was essentially compelled to return to Egypt to extricate the Children of Israel from bondage (a job he resisted in the first place), only to be initially rejected by them and by Pharaoh. He endured countless challenges and complaints from the people during the years in the desert, and led them to Sinai only to have them craft and worship a golden calf when they believed he was *one day* late in coming down from the mountain. Having done all of that in the service of God and his people, what was his reward? To be denied entry into the Holy Land.

One need not, however, rely on religious or biblical examples to realize the universality of personal challenges. Indeed, unfortunately, contemporary history is replete with examples of righteous people being handed seemingly unfair hardships. Take, for example, Raoul Wallenberg, the Swedish diplomat who issued protective passports and sheltered Jews from Nazi persecution, saving, in all likelihood, tens of thousands of lives, only to be imprisoned (and possibly executed) by the Soviets after the war.

Mr. Saltzman sits next to me each week in synagogue. He is a slight, sweet, gentle old man who never utters a negative word about anyone. When he reaches out to shake my hand the numbers tattooed on his arm are visible. He lived through *seven different concentration camps.* He lost many of his family members. He then went on to meet his wife in a displaced persons camp (she herself was kept alive throughout World War II because she was an opera singer and the Nazi officers made her perform for them). They came to America and built a life and a family. Then the same force of evil that persecuted them in their youth returned to haunt them again on September 11, 2001, when their son was murdered in the World Trade Center. Over the still-smoldering ruins of the Twin Towers, Mr. Saltzman turned to me and said, "This is the second time in my life that I have no grave to go to." If there was ever a person who had a right to be bitter and ask, "Why me? Why *always* me?" it is him. And yet, every person he meets is greeted with a smile and his twinkling eyes.

When I was in the hospital undergoing high-dose chemotherapy following my leukemia diagnosis, Danny, a doctor friend, came to visit me. Among the many things we discussed and the questions he asked me was, "Do you ever wonder, 'Why me'?" My immediate thought was of my dear friend Moshe. Moshe was, and continues to be, a pious person. He adheres to his faith, is charitable and has involved himself in his community. He served as a volunteer firefighter and served and led services in his synagogue. He walked miles to visit patients in the hospital on the high holidays and offered to blow the shofar (ram's horn, a Rosh Hashanah ritual), for them if they had been unable to hear it in synagogue. When one of his good friends, a landscaper, hurt his back, Moshe undertook to mow lawns and service all of his friend's clients, to keep his friend in business.

One Fourth of July weekend, Moshe's family was involved in a tragic fire. His mother-in-law was killed in the fire itself (the firefighters actually found her body huddled over two of his daughters, obviously trying to protect them). Moshe and two of his daughters were severely injured, with him suffering severe smoke damage to his lungs and his daughters suffering extensive burns. For some weeks the girls languished in the burn center of New York Hospital while many of us gathered in a continuous prayer vigil. Ultimately, the girls passed away, and their funerals were among the most horrible things I have ever experienced firsthand. Moshe's ordeal seemed, to me, to be entirely unfair.

However, when I went to see Moshe while he was sitting shiva (a weeklong ritual Jewish mourning period following the funeral of an immediate relative), he told me that he had to believe that what had happened was *l'tova*, a Hebrew expression meaning "for the best." When I asked him how he could think that way in the face of such an enormous tragedy, he explained that his family's tragedy, and the suffering of his daughters, led many people to perform incredible acts of kindness toward his family. They gathered in prayer and support, raised funds to offset the enormous costs of treatment, resettling, and replacing the property that they had lost and rallied to help Moshe and his family through the crisis. Because the fire had happened during the summer months, immediately before the Jewish high holidays of Rosh Hashanah and Yom Kippur (when Jews believe that they must repent for the past year's sins and a divine determination is made as to whether they will merit another year of life, and the quality of that year), Moshe told me that he believed that his daughters' plight helped many people "over the hump" for that year, by providing them the opportunity to perform tremendous acts of kindness that would outweigh any of their sins and earn them the merit for another good year.

Needless to say, his response had a very profound effect on me. While I know that this perspective was Moshe's means of self-preservation—that he was turning to his faith in God to cushion himself from the incomprehensible blow he had received—I never could have comprehended that someone could view such a horrendous circumstance in such a positive way.

So when Danny asked me if I wondered "Why me?" Moshe's response helped me find my "why." My own diagnosis occurred shortly before those same high holidays. My own friends and family rallied to my side, including me in their prayers (and spreading prayer requests literally worldwide over the Internet), cooking, shopping and baby-sitting for my family and coming to visit me often, bringing their good humor and trying to lift my spirits. I related Moshe's story to Danny and concluded simply that maybe it was just "my turn" to serve as the vehicle for others to multiply their righteous deeds before a time of judgment, and perhaps as well to give *them* added perspective as to their own good fortunes and the value of life. Indeed, several friends subsequently told me that, in the wake of my cancer, whenever they felt overwhelmed or overly focused on the difficulties of life, my situation helped them refocus on what is truly important in life and how most of life's "difficulties" are not as difficult as we ordinarily believe them to be.

If you too are struggling with "Why me?" ask yourself, as I did: "Am I really more pious than any of these people? Am I more entitled to a pain-free life? Is there something that makes me so special that I can feel legitimately that my cancer is somehow 'unfair'?" I think you will come to realize that cancer is neither fair to bad people nor unfair to good ones. It is neither your spiritual fault if you get it nor your spiritual right if you do not.

Rather, the unfortunate fact is that cancer has become ubiquitous in our society, where we are exposed, even unwittingly, to a variety of lifestyles and factors that have been determined to lead to cancer, whether they be environmental toxins, cigarette smoke, overconsumption of certain types of foods or work conditions. Further, although many cancers can be traced to lifestyle and environmental factors, genetics also can play a significant role. Stress, which compromises the immune system, is another possible culprit. In addition, due to advances in medical science and treatments for various illnesses that in times past led to deaths at a young age, people simply live longer now than they used to. Many types of cancer have particularly long latency periods and, as a result, the longer people live, the more likely it is that at some point they will be diagnosed with some form of cancer. These various factors have resulted in the fact that approximately *one out of every three* people will, at some point in their lives, be diagnosed with some form of cancer.[11]

Still, for some people, coming up with a "why?"—a reason on some spiritual or metaphysical level—helps lead to the acceptance of cancer. Asking yourself what your cancer may mean in terms of how you have lived your life, the effect of your disease on how you *continue* to live your life or how you prioritize life's many issues (whether they be how you handle money, talk to your children or spouse or stress too much over the "small stuff"), may help you find your "why." Bad things happen to all of us at one point or another. When life is proceeding according to the routines we all come to expect

---

11   The United States Department of Agriculture places the risk of cancer at some point in one's life at 41 percent. See "Dietary Guidelines for Americans, 2010," chapter 1, p. 3 (citing the National Cancer Institute, Surveillance Epidemiology and End Results (SEER) Stat Fact Sheets: All Sites; http://seer.cancer.gov/statfacts/html/all.html).

that thought is far from our minds. But coming to accept that fact—and that cancer may simply be *your* "bad thing"—can help you come to also accept, and therefore be better able to deal with, your cancer diagnosis.

Be Up, So You Won't Go Down for the Count

While for some people, no amount of self-reflection and soul searching will help them accept and come to grips with their diagnosis, for many cancer patients this reflection is critical. It can help alleviate the stress and depression that may accompany your diagnosis, and this may itself help in your recovery.

Indeed, some scientific studies—but by no means all studies investigating the issue—suggest that reducing depression and stress may be a critical factor in cancer survival. For example, one study noted that "[e]ighty-five percent of cancer patients and 71.4% of oncologists endorse the belief that psychological variables affect cancer progression."[12] This study indicated that:

> The current meta-analysis presents fairly consistent evidence that depression is a small but significant predictor of mortality in cancer patients. Estimates were as high as a 26% greater mortality rate among patients endorsing depressive symptoms and a 39% higher mortality rate among those diagnosed with major depression.[13]

---

12   See J. Satin, et al., "Depression as a Predictor of Disease Progression and Mortality in Cancer Patients: A Meta-Analysis," *Cancer*, 115, no. 22, 5349–5361 at 5349–5350, 5353–5354 (November 15, 2009) (the "Satin Study"). Dr. Satin and her colleagues analyzed more than thirty studies evaluating the effect of depression on the mortality rates of several thousand cancer patients.

13   Ibid., 5356.

Although the study authors noted some limitations in their analysis, they stated that it suggested that "depression may be an independent risk factor in cancer mortality, rather than merely correlating with biological factors associated with a poor prognosis."[14] The biological mechanism they suggested is an activation of the hypothalamopituitary-adrenal axis, which may affect the cellular immune system and thereby increase the potential for tumor growth. In addition, the authors noted that certain inflammatory molecules that play a role in the immune system can be affected adversely by depression.[15] In layman's terms, according to the Satin Study, depression may cause a biological response that inhibits the immune system and allows tumors to grow.[16] Thus, the study authors' analysis of the other studies that had been done on this issue suggests that depression by itself may be associated with whether someone survives cancer or not.

Another study associated depression among cancer patients with a twofold increase in the odds of dying from cancer.[17] The study authors concluded that their findings were "compatible with the hypothesis that psychological depression may be associated with impairment of mechanisms that prevent the establishment and spread of malignant cells."[18] In other words, their study suggests that depression may prevent the body from stopping the development and spread of cancer. Still other studies have shown that women suffering from breast and ovarian cancer had more effective natural killer cells when they maintained a high morale.[19]

---

14 Ibid.

15 Ibid., 5350.

16 Ibid.

17 R. B. Shekelle, et al., "Psychological Depression and 17-Year Risk of Death from Cancer," *Psychosom Med* (1981) 43:117–125 at 123–124.

18 Ibid., 124.

19 *Anticancer*, 143–144.

Not all studies have replicated such results and the effects of depression and psychological counseling on a patient's cancer survival continue to be studied and debated, however. Indeed, even studies that initially showed strong associations between reducing depression and long-term cancer survival rates showed a weaker, albeit still positive, association upon follow-up. For example, in a study evaluating the effects of group psychiatric counseling on survival rates among patients with malignant melanoma, the initial five- to six-year report on those patients showed that they had a significantly longer period of non-recurrence than patients who did not receive such counseling.[20] A follow-up study at ten years showed a slightly better, but no longer statistically significant, non-recurrence rate among the group that received counseling.[21]

In an initial study investigating the potential link between depression and mortality in breast cancer patients, supportive group therapy was associated with a survival advantage for the patients who utilized such therapy.[22] Although a ten-year follow-up on the participants in the study found that quality of life and pain reduction was higher in the therapy participants, long-term survival rates among the women receiving group support did *not* significantly exceed that of nonparticipants that far out.[23]

---

20 F. I. Fawzy, et al., "Effects of an Early Structured Psychiatric Intervention, Coping and Affective State on Recurrence and Survival 6 Years Later," *Arch Gen Psychiatry* (1993): 50: 681–689.

21 F. I. Fawzy, et al., "Malignant Melanoma: Effects of a Brief, Structured Psychiatric Intervention on Survival and Recurrence at 10-Year Follow-Up," *Arch Gen Psychiatry* (2003): 60: 100–103.

22 D. Spiegel, et al., "Effect of Psychosocial Treatment on Survival of Patients with Metastatic Breast Cancer," *Lancet* (1989): 2: 888–891.

23 G. Gellert, et al., "Survival of Breast Cancer Patients Receiving Adjunctive Psychosocial Support Therapy: A 10-Year Follow-Up Study," *Journal of Clinical Oncology* (1993):11: 66–69.

Thus, although there is some evidence that reducing depression and improving your mood may have actual physical benefits in terms of your ability to defeat your cancer, the full value of being "up" and remaining optimistic during the course of your cancer battle may lie in how an improved mood makes you *act*. When a person feels proactive about how he is dealing with his cancer and positive that what he is doing to defeat it—including things that are difficult—is going to work, he is more likely to make sure that he continues to follow his treatment protocol and try to otherwise do things to make himself feel better and increase the likelihood that his treatments will be successful. Indeed, even critics of psychological cancer treatment do note that such treatments can have non-clinical benefits:

> These techniques may reduce stress, alleviate depression, help control pain and enhance patients' feelings of mastery and control. Individual and group support can have a positive impact on quality of life and overall attitude. A positive attitude may increase a patient's chance of surviving cancer by increasing compliance with proven treatment.[24]

The bottom line is that, although virtually all cancer patients, including me, have moments of sadness or depression flowing from their illness or treatment (and you should not feel bad or blame yourself for sometimes feeling this way), becoming or staying depressed about your cancer may impede your recovery, either because it may compromise your ability to heal or discourage you from taking the steps necessary to do so. In contrast, the peace of mind that can flow from acceptance of a diagnosis and coming to grips with what has happened to you can foster the calm that will help you rise out

---

24 S. Barrett, "Questionable Cancer Therapies" ("Barrett"), available at http://www.quackwatch.com/01QuackeryRelatedTopics/cancer.html.

of any depressive funk, dissolve the stress you will undergo as you travel through your cancer treatment and help you accept what you have to do to defeat your disease, which in turn may help your body heal.

Which Doctor, Not Witch Doctor

For many cancer patients, the initial diagnosis or suspicion of cancer may not come from an oncologist, but rather from a general practitioner or other doctor who recognizes some type of irregularity (for example, a suspicious lump, irregular blood counts, an abnormal pap smear or some other type of symptom or indicator). As such, one of the most important decisions you will have to make early in your cancer journey is choosing an oncologist to shepherd you through your treatment. I say "choose" instead of "find" because determining which oncologist with whom to partner in your treatment is *your* choice. It can be a tough choice, because it can influence greatly the course of your treatment and how you feel along the way, but, like so many other cancer-related issues with which we contend, it need not be overwhelming.

There are several avenues to help you make your choice. You may, in fact, have been diagnosed definitively by an oncologist (probably one to whom you were referred by your primary care physician). If you trust your regular doctor's judgment and feel comfortable with the oncologist to whom he referred you, continuing to use that oncologist as your cancer doctor can be simple and convenient.

If you would like to investigate further—as is your right and is always a good idea—there are several paths to help you reach your goal:

- Family/friends: Because cancer has become so ubiquitous in our society, virtually everyone has family members or friends who have gone through it, either directly or through the illness of a loved one. If they had a positive relationship and experience with a particular oncologist, ask them to refer you to that doctor. Even if he is not a specialist in your particular type of cancer, he probably can refer you to someone who is.

- Your primary care doctor: The general practitioner you see regularly (or specialists with whom you may already have a relationship, such as a gynecologist or gastroenterologist) will likely be able to refer you to an oncologist she knows and trusts. If you trust your primary doctor's judgment, her recommendation may be a good starting point.

- Your insurance company: Most insurance companies maintain lists of specialists in your area who accept your insurance, which, for most people, is a significant issue, as the cost of cancer treatments can be astronomical, particularly if periods of hospitalization are required. Call your insurance carrier or visit its website to see which oncologists are available under your plan and where they are located. Then contact them, inquire as to their experience and set up a time to speak with and/or meet with them.

- Local hospital: Your local hospital (and other prominent hospitals) has affiliations with oncologists. If you call the hospital it should be able to supply you with contact information for those oncologists, and you can contact them to determine if they are the right doctor for you.

Moreover, in choosing an oncologist, keep in mind and inquire as to the following:

- Reputation: Is the oncologist you are considering a recognized specialist for the specific type and stage of cancer you have? If not, ask him to refer you to someone who is. Relevant to this consideration is how long he has been practicing in the particular specialty related to your condition. Ask, as well, if he has published scholarly articles in recognized publications or chairs or leads departments, or served on the board of recognized medical institutions or associations.

- Patient ratings: One of the advantages of today's online world is that the opinions of other people who have been in our situation often are readily available. If, for example, you run a search on Google for a doctor you are considering, you will come across sites on which patients rate doctors who have treated them. While these reviews are subjective and can be skewed by specific patients who may have clashed with that doctor, they can provide insight into issues that may be important to you in choosing your oncologist—including, for example, how available the doctor was to discuss patient concerns and open-mindedness toward complementary treatments. In addition, although doctors are bound by doctor-patient confidentiality requirements, a doctor you are considering may be able to refer you to other patients he or she has treated so that you can get a direct review from someone who actually has been treated by that doctor, perhaps for the same type of cancer you have.

- Personality: One of the most important factors in choosing your oncologist is whether you have a rapport with her. Ask yourself what personality traits are important to you in choosing your doctor. Do you want someone who is very gentle and will coddle you through your treatment? Do you want someone with a no-nonsense attitude who will always "give it to you straight" even if the news is difficult? Is open-mindedness toward complementary or alternative treatment methods important to you or are you satisfied with pursuing only conventional treatments? Do you want a doctor with a good sense of humor or is that unimportant as long as you have a doctor with the best reputation? Determine up front what your philosophy is in terms of what type of doctor you would respond to best, and then use that evaluation to help you choose an oncologist to treat you.

- Local or long-distance: Is the oncologist you are considering located reasonably close to where you live or will you have to travel several hours or even to another state to be treated by him? Depending on the type and stage of cancer that you have, and the rapport you develop with a particular oncologist, you may either be best served by or want to be treated in a particular facility or by a particular doctor who practices far away. If you and your family are satisfied that this is your best option, by all means pursue it. Bear in mind, however, that being separated by hundreds, if not thousands, of miles from much of your familial or friendly support systems and being taken out of your comfort zone can add additional psychological challenges to your cancer journey and involve the increased cost and physical burden of travel.

- Big or small: Some patients feel that being treated in the biggest, most well-known hospital, or by the doctor with the biggest reputation, must be the best way to go. While there certainly can be advantages to being treated in such facilities or by such doctors—the reputations of which generally are well-earned—including, for example, access to some of the leading doctors and latest treatment methods, there are potential disadvantages as well. For the bigger the hospital (or doctor), the greater the chance that you will be only one among the multitude of patients treated, with less individualized attention and focus. The larger or more famous cancer hospitals also often are the centers in which cancer studies are conducted and, as a result, you run the risk of being considered and treated as part of a larger research project (although that obviously depends on the doctor who treats you). These were among the reasons why I chose North Shore University Hospital, although I could have been treated in a larger hospital, like Memorial Sloan-Kettering Cancer Center in Manhattan. If, however, you gain peace of mind from knowing that you are being treated in a hospital or by a doctor of great renown and are convinced that you will receive the best care from him, by all means pursue that avenue of treatment.

- Insurance coverage: For most cancer patients, any doctor, even the "best" one, simply is not a viable choice if that doctor is not covered under the patient's insurance plan. Unless you have the financial wherewithal to engage an oncologist outside of your insurance coverage, find out first which ones *are* covered and reach out to them.

- Negative publicity or lawsuits: Online research also can indicate whether a doctor you are considering has been subject to lawsuits (either for malpractice or fraudulent claims regarding the efficacy of a treatment she may have developed and is promoting) or criticism within the established medical community (for example, whether she has been accused of "quackery" or promoting unproven or dangerous alternative treatments). While lawsuits sometimes have no basis (and merely being sued does not indicate any wrongdoing or liability), and criticism of a particular method does not necessarily exclude it, these types of information can give you pause as to whether to engage a certain doctor or at least provide you with areas of inquiry for that doctor.

My own referral to my oncologist came from my mother, and that doctor had treated my grandmother, so my family already had a relationship with him. He also was associated with North Shore University Hospital, which has a dedicated leukemia ward, a good reputation and has the added benefit of being close to where I live. It was also a place where I felt that I would not get "lost in the shuffle." When I met with him, I found him to be of good humor and he had a gentle way of dealing with me. Even when he gave me my diagnosis, he was truthful and straightforward but also realistically optimistic. I felt comfortable with him, and that really is the most important aspect of choosing your oncologist.

While obviously you need to make sure that the oncologist you choose has a good reputation and is associated with a good hospital, ultimately the "right" doctor has to be the right doctor *for you.* Even if you are referred to the "best" doctor in the field, she is only the "best" doctor *for you* if she is someone with whom you are infinitely comfortable and who meshes with your personality. Some people want an assertive doctor who will take charge and tell them what to do. Other people want a doctor who will act more like a partner in their care, exchanging ideas and being open-minded to other approaches. Many patients need a doctor with a comforting bedside manner, whereas for others that aspect is irrelevant as long as the doctor can heal them.

You should endeavor to choose an oncologist with whom you are most comfortable and who will give you the time and attention you need. Choose someone who will not only point you in the right direction but walk the path to your goal *with you*; someone who will advocate for you, be there when you need him and coordinate your care both as an inpatient and an outpatient to make sure that all of your treating physicians or other health-care providers (including complementary medical practitioners) are on the same page. Do your due diligence in seeking out an oncologist, and then factor into your decision whether a particular oncologist fits into how you want and need to be treated.

CHAPTER 3

GETTING THE INFORMATION

*"A man's life in these parts often depends
on a mere scrap of information."*
Clint Eastwood, *A Fistful of Dollars*

Once you have dealt with the shock of your initial diagnosis and the pressing issues of letting people know what is going on with you and choosing your oncologist, you will probably, like a lot of cancer patients, want to learn about your disease and treatment, and you should learn as much as possible. Getting the right information is crucial to understanding what is happening with your body, what likely *will* happen to it and what your treatment will entail.

Just Ask

Your oncologist should be the primary source of your information. He should spend as much time with you as necessary for you to get the information you need. Do not be afraid of pressing him or pursuing the answers you want. Do not think that the questions you ask are too silly or trivial. *You* are the one with cancer. *You* are the one who will be undergoing treatment. You have the right to ask whatever you want. Bear in mind, however, that your doctor has a lot of other patients and may not always be available exactly when you want him.

An efficient approach is to make a list of all of the questions you have so that you can get them all addressed when you have your doctor's attention.

Indeed, when I got my own diagnosis and I had finished asking my questions, my doctor asked if we had any more. My wife asked simply, "Are you sure he has leukemia?" That was a question many people might think is too presumptuous to ask. They might feel uncomfortable about challenging their doctor's diagnosis. But my doctor simply chuckled and said, "That's a very good question. Yes, I ran the results past several of my colleagues and they confirmed my diagnosis." My wife, still unsatisfied, spoke to her brother (who is an OB/GYN with a subspecialty in oncology), and he in turn asked for copies of the slides my doctor had taken of my bone marrow so he could look at them himself. My doctor had no problem with that, and sent them along.

Your doctor should be equally willing to be questioned or even challenged. As discussed elsewhere in this book, second opinions are common and, before you undertake an onerous course of treatment, it makes all the sense in the world to get one. That second opinion can cover not only the diagnosis itself but the treatment options as well. If your doctor has told you that you need surgery, another doctor may feel it is unnecessary, or that a less radical surgery is possible, which itself might make your treatment and recovery less painful and shorter. One doctor may tell you that you need to undergo chemotherapy, whereas another might feel that radiation is the proper way to go. Or another doctor may simply believe that your condition does not need immediate, radical treatment. The point is, you should control how far the discussions about your cancer and its treatment go, and let the medical professionals address for you what ultimately is the best course of treatment. Once that is done, you will have a greater level of comfort that the course of treatment you have chosen in consultation with your doctors is the best one.

To help you get started, the following are some of the questions you may want to ask your doctor, keeping in mind, of course, that each person will have specific questions that relate more directly to him based on his own situation:

- What is the exact type and stage of cancer that I have? Understanding specifically what type of cancer you have and how far it has progressed is critical to your understanding of what type of treatment is going to be required and why and how that treatment is likely to affect you.

- What are my options for treatment? Along these same lines, you may want to ask what the most common treatment for your specific cancer/stage is and how effective it has been shown to be.

- If your doctor recommends surgery, are there approaches to your surgery that may be less invasive yet equally effective?

- Are there any complementary treatments (other than standard chemotherapy, radiation or surgical treatments) that have shown promise in treating my cancer? If so, what are the potential risks of those treatments?

- Am I eligible to participate in any clinical trials that may improve my chances of success or may enhance my regular course of treatment?

- Will I need to be hospitalized or can I be treated as an outpatient? If you need to be hospitalized, ask how long that hospitalization is likely to last and whether your doctor will be checking on you regularly when you are in the hospital.

- What are the potential side effects of the medication I will need to take or treatments I will be receiving? Will those effects be long-lasting or short-term? Do I need to do anything to address those side effects before or during my treatment (for example, storing eggs or sperm in case your treatment affects fertility)?

- Will I have physical limitations as a result of my treatment that will prevent me from working or performing activities of daily living (for example, getting dressed, showering, toileting) such that I will need to arrange to have someone available to assist me in those things or alert my employer that I will be out of work for a while?

- Does your doctor consult with a team of other doctors so that someone will always be available to answer your questions or concerns if your doctor is unavailable at some point during your treatment?

Getting these basic questions answered before you start your treatment will give you a basis for understanding what to expect as you begin your treatment and perhaps an enhanced feeling of control over your situation, while (hopefully) not bombarding you with too much information to absorb effectively.

The Internet: A Valuable but Dangerous Resource

The times have also changed. There was a time when the avenues for making informed inquiries about your condition, or the notion of challenging a doctor's diagnosis, did not exist. Informed consent in those days meant, for the most part, simply accepting whatever you were told by your doctor. That time has passed. The Internet has, simply and completely, altered the notion of informed consent. Now, you have literally at your fingertips access to a wellspring of information about your particular condition and the potential treatments for it. Whatever cancer you have, there are websites, blogs, chat rooms and support groups available online for you to tap into. Groups have been set up on social networking sites like Facebook as well. It can be a wonderful thing, as you can get information, advice and encouragement from all over the world. You can find people who have been exactly where you are and can help shepherd you through the process. Internet research is also a great way to become more versed in and more comfortable with some of the medical terminology relevant to your disease and treatment options, so that when you hear or see those terms you will be familiar with them.

But beware: There is such a thing as information overload. You will only be able to process so much information at once, although you will probably have a desire to get as much information as possible. Before embarking on an Internet search for answers, make a list of the issues you really want to know about and will want to address with your doctor, as discussed above. For example:

- What will probably happen to my body?
- How are people affected by the drugs I will take or other treatments I will undergo?
- What can I do to lessen those effects?
- What are the options for other treatments?
- What are some of the groups I can turn to for support?
- What are my rights in terms of my treatment? (Some of these basic rights are discussed in chapter 5.)
- What are my rights in connection with my job and missing time for treatment (particularly if you are going to be out of work for an extended period of time)? (Some of these rights are discussed in chapter 4.)

Try to stick to the basics as much as possible. You will hopefully have plenty of time to research further issues regarding your condition and prognosis going forward.

Be aware also that some websites are more reliable than others. In general, sites associated with major hospitals, universities or recognized medical organizations (the American

Cancer Society, the American Medical Association, the National Cancer Institute, the University of Pennsylvania Abramson Cancer Center link—www.oncolink.upenn.edu, etc.) will have more reliable information. The Internet is still an unregulated place in terms of the accuracy of information random individuals can post, and much of what you will find on unregulated or unsupervised websites or blogs will promote unproven cures or techniques for dealing with cancer. The information you may find on some of those sites may be inaccurate or even dangerous. That does not mean, however, that you should not ask your doctor about any information you find that may be relevant to your treatment (in fact, you may want to put together some files on some of the issues you come across to specifically review with your doctor), but non-professionals may simply not have access to the best or most updated information on a disease or its treatment.[25]

Strive to Fail Statistics

I would also caution you against focusing too much on the "statistics" of your particular cancer. I understand firsthand how much cancer patients "live by the numbers." We all want to know what the numbers tell us in terms of the likelihood of our survival. On the one hand, a high percentage survival rate for your cancer can be very encouraging. It is very easy, however, to get caught up in survival rates and what "your chances" are, and no matter how good the survival rates are in reported studies, there will be some percentage of people who do not survive, and it may be hard for you to ignore that

---

25   For a more thorough discussion of how to utilize the Internet in connection with your cancer diagnosis and potential treatments, see A. Schorr and M. Thomas, *The Web-Savvy Patient: An Insider's Guide to Navigating the Internet When Facing Medical Crisis.*

possibility. In my own case, my doctor told me that the cure rate for my type of leukemia was approximately 70 percent. While that was an encouraging number, the inescapable fact was that that meant that three out of every ten people who got my disease died, and it was hard to get that thought out of my head.

If you do investigate the survival rates (and I know you will), bear in mind that every individual is different. There simply is no mathematical formula for survival that can be applied accurately to everyone suffering from a particular form of cancer. For many reasons, one person's cancer may be more resilient than another's. One patient may be in better overall health than patients who have been studied and who have not survived. Some of the survival rates you will see may be based on studies that were done some years ago, before certain advances in treating your type of cancer. Even factors that have often gone largely unmeasured in studies on cancer mortality—including, for example, a patient's emotional support system and mental attitude—may significantly affect any one person's ability to withstand treatments and conquer his disease. Moreover, the statistics regarding cancer survival rates often simply do not take into account differences between patients who embrace lifestyle changes (such as following a healthier diet, exercise and stress management) and patients who continue in their potentially cancer-promoting lifestyles (such as continuing to eat a poor diet or smoke, or persist in a sedentary lifestyle). As such, the statistics are often skewed by people who simply do not do everything they can to beat their cancer. *You* will not make those mistakes.

Indeed, there are people who have survived even the most challenging, seemingly terminal cancers (including, for example, pancreatic, bone, bladder, ovarian and lung cancers) notwithstanding daunting recovery statistics. Among these was noted evolutionary scientist Stephen Gould. Gould was diagnosed with abdominal mesothelioma, an "incurable" condition with a median survival time of approximately eight months. Gould, however, lived *twenty years*—some thirty times longer than his initial prognosis—and died of an unrelated disease.[26]

In *Anticancer*, Dr. Servan-Schreiber describes the remarkable case of Ian Gawler, a veterinarian who was diagnosed with seemingly terminal bone cancer. When conventional cancer treatments failed to stop the spread of his cancer, Dr. Gawler undertook a regimen of intensive meditation—coupled with a natural diet and other natural treatments—and overcame a seemingly undefeatable cancer.[27]

Then there is Chris Calaprice. Calaprice, a former army ranger, was diagnosed with pancreatic cancer in 2003. He underwent chemotherapy and beat his cancer, only to have it recur a couple of years later. He underwent another round of chemotherapy and has survived for almost another decade. He also has gone through a bout with melanoma. In fact, he has undertaken a motorcycle journey covering more than forty-three thousand miles to help raise awareness and funds for pancreatic cancer research.[28] Supreme Court Justice Ruth Bader Ginsberg underwent surgery for pancreatic cancer in 2009, heard arguments twelve days after her surgery and continues to serve on the Court.

Thus, regardless of what "the numbers" say, resolve to avail yourself of the things discussed elsewhere in this book that

---

26 Gould's perspective on the inapplicability of statistics in cancer prognoses can be found in his excellent short article, "The Median Isn't the Message," available at http://cancerguide.org/median_not_msg.html.

27 *Anticancer*, 137–138.

28 See a description of Calaprice's incredible and inspiring journey at http://www.motorcycle-usa.com/653/8507/Motorcycle-Article/Chris-Calaprices-42-000-Mile-Road-2-A-Cure.aspx.

will give you an edge in overcoming your cancer, including proper nutrition and relaxation techniques that will help you reduce the stress attendant to having cancer and undergoing treatment. Resolve to live. Doing those things may help you distinguish your outcome from the percentage of people who are unable to overcome their cancers.

Good Intentions, Bad Information

Another double-edged sword in terms of getting information is the many well-meaning friends and relatives who will rush to your aid. Invariably, they will bring their own experiences and stories of people they have known who went through cancer and either lived through it or did not. The fact is that many people simply do not know what to say to someone who has cancer, due to their own discomfort or inexperience. Moreover, even other people who have gone through cancer themselves, or know other people who have, may be basing their knowledge on a cancer different in type or scope than yours. They may have gone through different treatments than you are undergoing or may have gone through such treatments a long time ago. As such, their experiences or the stories they relate may have absolutely no relevance to your own situation. Much has been accomplished in recent years in terms of cancer treatment and survival that simply did not exist years ago. As a result, the people you know may provide information and say things or tell stories that are unhelpful, discouraging or even obsolete.

For example, APL—the type of leukemia I had—was first diagnosed in the late 1950s and, in the ensuing two decades, there was no effective treatment. It was essentially 100 percent fatal. Had I discussed my cancer with someone whose only experience with APL was twenty years old, the doom-and-gloom story they would have related would have been entirely irrelevant (but I might not have known that). Try to absorb the good, encouraging information these people bring you and let any of the bad stuff slide past you. Welcome their support and love while tuning out anything negative.

CHAPTER 4

"WORK"ING IT OUT

"I'm just a little worried about my future."
Dustin Hoffman, *The Graduate*

As if cancer patients did not have enough to deal with just absorbing the reality of their diagnosis, deciding on a course of treatment and then going through it, cancer—especially when it will involve extended absence from work—raises the specter of financial uncertainty. While each person's work situation is different—and many people have understanding employers that will preserve a position notwithstanding a lengthy cancer-related absence, simply because it is the right thing to do—it is important to know your rights in terms of protecting your job.

First, if your job provides disability benefits, immediately upon being diagnosed contact the person who administers that disability program. Even if you do not yet know what your course of treatment will be or how long you will be out of work, alerting your employer to the probability that you will be out of work for a while and getting the ball rolling in terms of forms that need to be filled out to begin your disability coverage are important steps toward lessening your burden when you begin treatment. Your oncologist will be able to fill out relevant portions of those forms for your employer to make sure that you receive your disability benefits. Keep copies of any forms you fill out or receive from your employer, doctor or disability carrier in a "disability file."

There are also certain federal laws that may provide an amount of protection for your job position while you are sick or undergoing treatment, provided that you meet the requirements of those laws. Foremost among these is the Family and Medical Leave Act of 1993 (FMLA). Under the FMLA, an employee who (i) has been employed with an employer for at least 12 months, and (ii) worked at least 1,250 hours for that employer during the 12-month period immediately preceding the leave taken for illness, and (iii) works for an entity with at least 50 employees (either at the same location or within 75 miles of where the sick employee works) is considered an "eligible employee" for coverage under the FMLA.

An eligible employee is entitled to up to a total of 12 work weeks of unpaid leave during any 12-month period, either because the employee herself is unable to work because of a "serious health condition" that prevents her from performing, or interferes with her ability to perform, her job duties or must care for an immediate family member (a spouse, child or parent) who has a serious health condition. A "serious health condition" under the FMLA includes an illness, injury, impairment or physical or mental condition that involves (i) inpatient care in a hospital, hospice or residential care community, or (ii) continuing treatment by a health care provider. Most types of cancer would likely fit under these criteria. While the 12 weeks of leave need not be taken in one block, you may be required to provide the requisite statutory notice and provide re-certification to your employer that leave is required and meets the FMLA criteria each time you take another leave.

Although an employee ordinarily is required to give thirty days' advance notice before taking a leave under the FMLA, this requirement may be waived in an emergent situation, for example when you have been diagnosed with cancer and must begin treatment in less than thirty days. You must provide your employer with enough information for it to determine that you are, in fact, eligible for leave under the FMLA. A letter from your oncologist setting out your diagnosis and treatment plan, or copies of the tests that determined that you have cancer, may be sufficient for your employer's needs. Make sure to clarify with your employer exactly what information it needs and provide it with that information as soon as possible.

One of the primary benefits of the FMLA is that it protects the job of the person who takes leave under its terms. When you return to work, you have a right to be restored to your original job or an equivalent position. In other words, you cannot be fired or demoted if you take a leave that is authorized under the FMLA.

Another federal statutory scheme that may protect your rights at work is the Americans with Disabilities Act (ADA). The ADA makes it illegal for employers to discriminate against persons who have certain types of disabilities; namely physical (or mental) impairments that substantially limit the person's "major life activities" (sometimes referred to as activities of daily living), including, for example, walking, talking, seeing or learning. Some typical examples of the types of impairments that would be covered under the ADA are being confined to or needing a wheelchair, reliance on assistive devices like canes and walkers, blindness or vision impairment and hearing loss. Depending on the type of cancer you have, or the treatment (for example, surgery) that you undergo, you may find yourself reliant on these types of devices or suffering from these types or impairments.

Under the ADA, employers with at least fifteen employees must provide individuals who qualify under the ADA's terms with an equal opportunity to benefit from all employment-related opportunities that would be available to other, non-disabled employees. These include opportunities for promotion and raises. In addition, employers must make "reasonable accommodations" for a person who suffers from covered disabilities (for example, by allowing that person to work remotely if the job description is conducive to such work and providing access to work areas sufficient to accommodate a disabled person's assistive devices, such as wheelchair access).

Employers (particularly state and local governmental entities), however, may not be required to make accommodations that create substantial financial or administrative burdens, or otherwise would fundamentally affect the nature of the services or products they provide. For example, a company that provides armed guards whose job it is to protect employees or assets would not be required to hire, or revise its standards to accommodate, someone with the impairments listed above, because doing so would render the company incapable of providing adequately the service for which it is hired. Bear in mind that each state may also have laws affecting or protecting your rights in connection with your job during your cancer treatment, and you should consult with an employment lawyer in your home state to make sure that you get the protection the law provides.

Even if you do not qualify for protection under the FMLA or the ADA, your protection at work may be assured by your employer itself. If you have a close enough relationship with your employer or have been an employee for a long period of time, your employer may simply decide that you can take an extended leave for your cancer treatment and return to your position. While most employees are "at will," which means that they can be fired at any time for any non-discriminatory reason, and therefore any informal assurance from your employer that your position is safe would probably not be legally binding, having the assurances of someone for whom you have worked for many years or with whom you have developed a close personal, as well as professional, relationship, can go a long way toward easing some of your concerns. Be up front and honest with your employer as soon as you have an idea of what your cancer and its treatment will entail, and update them regularly as to your progress. This will help cement the feeling of trust running between you and your employer as you go through your treatment.

In my own case, I was fortunate to work for a firm that has a good disability policy, which covered a substantial portion of my salary during my almost year-long absence. I also had what I consider to have been even more important to my peace of mind and ultimate recovery, however: the support of those with whom and for whom I worked. On the day I got my diagnosis, one of the first calls I made (after my family members) was to the senior partner of my law firm. When his secretary told me he was busy, I insisted and told her that it was important that I speak with him. Initially, he picked up my call on speakerphone, which indicated to me that, as usual, he was in the middle of something, but as soon as I told him that I had leukemia he picked up the phone and spoke to me with genuine concern, offering to help get me into Sloan-Kettering if I wanted and throwing his personal support, and the support of the firm, behind me.

My other colleagues similarly offered both me and my wife their encouragement and support throughout my hospitalization and treatment. Indeed, when I first returned to visit the firm after my release from the hospital, with my newly bald head, the senior partner (my boss), broke into tears and hugged me, telling me how wonderful it was to see me. Other colleagues expressed similar sentiments. That kind of support helped nurture me through my ordeal and, in fact, made me an even more dedicated employee when I returned to work. The rapport and relationships you have built over the years with the people with whom you work may provide you with the same type of support and encouragement.

CHAPTER 5

STARTING YOUR TREATMENT

"Start by doing what's necessary; then do what is possible; and suddenly you are doing the impossible."

Francis of Assisi

When someone is diagnosed with cancer, the immediate, natural reaction on their part is to want to start treatment as soon as possible. We are so emotionally repulsed by the very idea of having cancer that the knee-jerk reaction is to "get it out" or get it treated *right now*. Indeed, because a cancer diagnosis is usually followed by a flurry of activity, including follow-up appointments, second opinions, phone calls to relatives and friends and intense investigation of your condition, the overall sense of urgency can be heightened.

Bear in mind, however, that, at least for several types of cancer, you may not need to start your treatment immediately. Many cancers, especially tumorigenic cancers, develop over many months or even years. In fact, many people discover their cancers "accidentally," while undergoing a routine examination or running their hand casually over a part of their body and noticing an unusual lump. Accordingly, for those types of cancers, a slight delay in treatment will probably not materially affect your prognosis or chances for survival. While obviously you will not want to delay your treatment for very long (and in some circumstances, such as my own, treatment may need to begin as soon as possible), you may very well have some time to collect your thoughts and plan your course of action.

As a general rule of thumb, be "QUICK": (i) question; (ii) understand; (iii) investigate; (iv) challenge; and (v) keep informed.

Question

As discussed above, it is incumbent upon you to ask all of the questions you want regarding the nature of your disease, potential treatment methods (both conventional and alternative) and your prognosis. No question is too silly or inconsequential, and your doctor should entertain them all. Do not ever feel embarrassed to ask any question. As the Chinese proverb advises, "He who asks a question is a fool for five minutes; but he who does not ask is a fool forever."

If you are presented with a treatment option, ask how the treatment will likely affect you. What are the potential immediate side effects? What are the potential long-term adverse effects (including secondary cancers, reproductive effects or other chronic disorders)? While chemotherapy or radiation may be an important part of your victory over cancer, the fact is that those treatments themselves are extremely toxic and can cause secondary cancers down the road. Truly, if you did not have cancer, you would never dream of purposely exposing yourself to the agents involved in these treatments.

If your cancer is particularly advanced, you may want to ask frank questions about how different your quality of life will be with the treatment as opposed to not undergoing it at all. For some advanced cancer patients, chemotherapy, radiation or surgery may only prolong life for a period of weeks, yet they undergo onerous treatments that leave them sick or debilitated for what little time they gain. For those patients, not undergoing any of these conventional treatments may actually be a better approach. The fact that your doctor suggests a particular course of treatment may make it seem like that is the only or preferred course, but that is often simply not the case, and you should ask your doctor and other consulting doctors what other treatment options exist. As discussed in chapter 15, those options include alternative or complementary therapies to chemotherapy, radiation and surgery.

The overriding question you need to ask yourself and others involved in your care (including those closest to you who will have to live with and shepherd you through the course of treatment you choose) is: What is the best course of treatment *for me*? Most of us have been raised to consider selfishness a vice to be avoided. When you are deciding how to fight your cancer, however, selfishness is both acceptable and necessary. It is *your* body. It is *your* life. The decision as to which path to take, or whether and how to combine different approaches, ultimately is *your* decision, not anyone else's.

Viewed in this light, your decision to get a second (or third or fourth) opinion is perfectly acceptable, even if you have already seen "the best" doctor in the field. Your second opinion should be from a doctor who is unaffiliated with the doctor who diagnosed you, and I encourage you to bring along someone whose opinion you value or who can function as a strong advocate for your interests. If you have a relative or friend who is herself a doctor, even an oncologist, ask her to accompany you on your visit to the doctor so you can have someone there who can better gauge whether you are getting the right and complete information.

In addition, because this will be a time when you are inundated with information—much of which will be in language you have never encountered and may not understand—keep track of what you are told. Take notes or have someone who accompanies you do so. Recording your conversations with doctors and others is a convenient and sensible method with which to keep track of and understand critical information. It will prevent you from forgetting what is important and allow you to listen to and review it later to make sure that you have all of the information you need and understand what you have been told.[29]

Understand

Before and during your treatment, a lot of information will be thrown your way. Never feel embarrassed about asking for a clearer explanation of the information given to you. If the second explanation is still confusing or vague, ask for it to be clarified even further. Unless you are a doctor or other medical professional, you probably have little experience dealing with medical terms or understanding how certain treatments will affect you biologically or psychologically. There is no shame in this. In fact, even doctors who do not specialize in oncology may be ignorant of or not fully understand everything involved with cancer prognosis and treatment. Many specialized oncologists, in contrast, are so well versed in the "medicalese" of your condition and treatment that they may express themselves or explain things to you in a manner that is simply over your head because you are not used to dealing with the terms involved in understanding your condition or treatment. Understanding clearly the nature of your cancer and the treatments you will be receiving will help you make an informed decision about what you are going to be doing (or refusing to do) to your body.

---

29 Bear in mind, however, that, in some states, it may be illegal to record a conversation unless the person being recorded knows she is being recorded, so let your doctor or other people with whom you are consulting know that you want to record your conversations with them before you do so. Few doctors or other health-care providers will object to you doing so.

When I was admitted to the hospital the day after my diagnosis, I was presented with a myriad of forms to sign that related to my treatment and the terms of my hospital stay. The administrators who gave them to me stood by, waiting for me to sign them and hand them back, as I am sure almost all patients do, without really reading them. When I began to read each document thoroughly, one of them said, "You must be a lawyer, because no one else actually reads these things." That was accurate, of course, and, being the uptight lawyer that I am, I would counsel a client never to sign a document relating to his rights without reading it carefully first and making sure he understood it, so I for sure was not going to sign anything that related to my own treatment without reading it carefully and asking whatever questions I had.

My experience as a toxic tort (chemical exposure) and product liability lawyer gave me the tools to pick apart and understand much of the technical jargon involved with my condition and treatment and the skills to investigate the science involved in making my treatment decisions. I know that most people do not have that background and that going through the multipage documents you are handed is probably the last thing you want to do, but remember that the documents you sign define your rights as a patient and include vital information about the type of treatment you will receive. Read them carefully. If necessary to your full understanding of what you will be going through, ask your doctor or a hospital administrator to go through them with you.

In my own case, I asked some very pointed questions about what I read: What if I did not want to undergo parts of my treatment? Would the information collected about my case be shared with others? What eligibility did I have to participate in clinical trials that might improve my chances for survival? What effect would the chemotherapy drugs have on me, both short-term and long-term? Were those drugs genotoxic (in other words, was there any science showing that the drugs I would be given could damage my genes in a way that could cause secondary cancers)? There were actually some provisions about waiving any liability against the hospital if someone was grossly negligent in my care that I objected to strongly and actually crossed out of the documents. When the hospital raised an objection, I stuck to my guns and revised some of the language to assuage my concerns and satisfy the hospital.

Bear in mind, however, that while the hospital or your doctor may be somewhat flexible, much of what is contained in these forms is "standard" language that has evolved and been compiled over the course of many hours by doctors, hospitals, federal or state regulatory agencies and lawyers. As such, there will be many provisions that are not subject to modification, and raising too many objections or refusing ultimately to sign the hospital's or doctor's forms may disqualify you from a life-saving treatment or study. The bottom line is, if you see something in the information given to you or the forms you are directed to sign that either confuses or concerns you, raise it and see if it can be explained or resolved to your satisfaction. Understanding what you are agreeing to and what will happen to you as a result *is your right*. Insist upon it, but never lose sight of the ultimate goal: getting the treatment you need.

Investigate

Once you know how your doctor is proposing to treat your cancer, you can—and should —investigate thoroughly what the proposed treatment will entail. In this regard, you can employ some of the approaches discussed in chapters 1, 2 and 3, to wit: (i) get your second opinion on the course of treatment you are considering (and third and fourth opinions, if necessary); (ii) talk to others who have undergone that treatment to see how it affected them; (iii) go to your local library and ask the librarian to direct you to some resources that may be informative; and (iv) use the Internet wisely to locate information and support groups to help guide you. If you do not know anyone personally who has gone through the particular treatment you are going to undergo, ask your doctor or the hospital to direct you to someone.

Many cancer patients are more than happy to give guidance and support to their comrades in arms. In addition, just as soldiers often express how only another soldier who has seen combat can relate to what it is like, only another cancer patient can truly relate to what it is like to endure chemotherapy, radiation or other cancer treatments. A firsthand perspective from our side of the bedrail is an indispensable asset both in determining what treatment plan to undertake and understanding the effects that treatment will entail. Moreover, speaking to people who have been where you are and have emerged out the other side can provide you with enormous encouragement as to your ability to defeat your own cancer.

Further, if your treatment will require hospitalization, inquire as to the reputation and facilities of that hospital. There are hospital rating guides available online, which can provide a candid review of the strengths and weaknesses of different hospitals. Some of those reviews will come from professional organizations and look at the overall quality of the hospital and doctors employed there, including specific departments within the hospital.[30] Others are composed of patient reviews and can give you a perspective that may be more directly relevant to you (for example, by discussing from the patient's view the attentiveness of the hospital staff,

---

30 *U.S. News & World Report* has a comprehensive ranking of hospitals nationwide, by specialty and geographical location. It is available at http://health.usnews.com/best-hospitals.

cleanliness, comfort, facilities for visitors, etc.).[31] Especially if you are going to be hospitalized repeatedly or for an extended period of time, you need to be comfortable with what your inpatient experience will be like.

Challenge

For many people, the concept of challenging their doctors is alien. Perhaps they were raised to respect doctors and grew up during a time when if your doctor told you to do something, you did it. Some people simply want to avoid confrontation, and this may be particularly true when you feel the effects of your cancer or treatments. Being willing to challenge either what you are told or what is being done to you, however, is a vital skill. *Be proactive.* Again, for better or for worse, it is *your cancer.* It is *your treatment.* It is *your body.* It is *your life.* If something is causing you physical or emotional distress, ask if there is something else you can do.

For example, if, like many cancer patients, you are experiencing gastrointestinal problems (nausea, vomiting, diarrhea, constipation) from your chemotherapy or radiation, and the anti-nausea or other drugs you are being given to counteract these effects are not working, ask for something else. Thankfully, there are many drugs available today that can alleviate these effects, and not all drugs that work for one person will work for another. If you are in pain, and the medicine that is being given to you to reduce that pain is insufficient, ask whether your dosage can be increased or if there is another pain medication that you can use. Perhaps you are a candidate for self-administered pain medication, which will allow you to administer doses to yourself without having to wait for a nurse to respond to your call. There may

---

31 See, for example, some of the reports located at http://consumer-healthratings.com.

be another approach that will help you get through your treatments than the one you are using. There is no need for you to "suffer in silence." Let your bravado stand aside and ask for something that will help you.

Also, if, for some reason, you decide that you do not want to take certain medications, or want to stop a particular medication, say so. No one can force you to take something you do not want to take. Make sure, however, that your decision is a sound one that considers your doctor's input. I remember, for example, several incidents that occurred during my prolonged hospitalization. As a result of my leukemia and chemotherapy, my potassium levels were dangerously low, so I was put on an intravenous potassium drip. Anyone who has ever had a potassium drip knows that it burns terribly as the medicine is administered. I complained to the nurse, who diluted the IV. It still burned, however, and I was very uncomfortable. I asked whether I could just take a potassium supplement orally, as I was sure I had seen such supplements on the shelf of my local pharmacy. "Well, the pill you would have to take is really big," I was told. "Look," I said, "unless you have to shoot it into the back of my throat like you do with a horse, I'll get it down. Just get this damn thing out of my arm!" I got the pills.

Also during my hospitalization, I began running very high fevers. As a result, I was given amphotericin. For anyone unfamiliar with this particular antibiotic, it has been used to treat fungal infections and is sometimes given to patients when their fevers cannot be traced to any other source (although its use is less common now than when I was treated). It is noxious. It can damage your kidneys and heart. It can cause particularly bad rigor (intense shaking), so bad that the nurse put up my bedrails to prevent me from shaking myself out of bed. It is photosensitive and is delivered in a brown covering to prevent it from reacting to light. In plain terms, it is nasty—so nasty, in fact, that one of the nurses sat in my room while it was administered. Thankfully, I got through the administration of the amphotericin without incident.

Some days later, however, as my fevers had not subsided, the nurse came in with another dose. "What's that?" I asked.

"Amphotericin," she said.

"Isn't that for a fungal infection?" I asked.

"Yes," she said.

"Well, do I *have* a fungal infection?" I persisted.

"No," she said, "but since we don't know for sure what's causing your fever we are going to give you another dose."

Now, having been better informed about amphotericin since the first dose, I told her that I did not want it. She insisted at first, but I was adamant. "Look, if the infectious disease doctor comes in and tells me that I have to have it, I will consider it. Otherwise I am not taking it." I did not wind up taking the second dose.

On another occasion, after I had been discharged from the hospital but while I was still undergoing chemotherapy, I started to run a fever. As a result, my protocol required that I go to the emergency room. The attending doctor ran a series of blood tests and cultures and I waited at length for the results. At one point he came in with a hospital gown and told me to change into it. When I asked why, he told me that they would likely be admitting me to the hospital. After having spent a month there, that was the last thing I wanted.

"Are my blood results back yet?" I asked.

"No," he said, "but we may want to watch you for a couple of days," he told me.

"Well," I answered, "unless my blood comes back abnormal, you can watch my ass walking right out of this place." My blood came back okay, and I did not wind up staying in the hospital.

Indeed, most hospitals and doctors' offices will have a "Patient's Bill of Rights" (and such bills of rights may be dictated by individual state laws). Your rights as a patient may be described in such a policy. Ask your hospital or doctor if they have such a policy and, if so, ask for a copy of it. Typical provisions in such policies include your rights to:

- Full information regarding your health-care facility or doctor;
- Have someone address your questions in terms you can understand or, if you do not speak English, in your native language;
- Choose health-care providers who can give you high-quality health care when you need it;
- Know and understand your treatment options and make decisions about your care. You have the right to information about the benefits or side effects of a proposed treatment and the right to decline any particular treatment;
- Appoint a representative to make medical decisions for you if you cannot do so;
- Respectful, considerate and non-discriminatory care from the doctors, nurses and other health-care professionals who treat you;
- Confidentiality regarding your medical information (provided, however, that you may need to consent to the sharing of information among different doctors or facilities that treat you, in order to ensure that each doctor or facility has your full medical information and does not undertake any treatment that may be contraindicated for your condition);
- Read and copy your medical file (this can be especially important if you need or want to change doctors or hospitals);

• Have any complaints regarding your doctor, hospital or care reviewed fairly and in a timely manner.[32]

While I am not suggesting that you refuse to undergo any treatments simply because they may be dangerous or uncomfortable, I do encourage you to make your position known and insist on any concerns you have being resolved. You may ultimately decide to undergo a treatment even if you are concerned about its effects, but you are entitled to make that decision from a fully informed basis and after having had your concerns addressed. If, like me, you decide that certain aspects of your treatment simply are not for you, stand your ground. Do not let anyone (nurses, doctors or even your loved ones) bully you into a treatment that you, with full information, reject.

Keep Informed

Being properly informed about your cancer and how to defeat it does not end when you begin your treatment. Cancer treatment is an evolutionary process. It may depend on how you react to the treatment and whether the treatment is having its desired impact on your cancer (i.e., is it working). While many cancer treatment regimens are somewhat like the stock market, inasmuch as daily fluctuations do not necessarily reflect the bigger picture, you should ask for regular updates on your lab results and how the treatment is progressing. Keep your own file of the medical and lab reports you receive. If things are not going as you had hoped or expected, discuss these issues with your doctor. Some treatments just take longer to take effect than others or than we may hope.

---

32 See, e.g., American Cancer Society, "Patient's Bill of Rights: What is the Patient's Bill of Rights," available at http://www.cancer.org/Treatment/FindingandPayingforTreatment/UnderstandingFinancialandLegal-Matters/patients-bill-of-rights.

Further, if your cancer treatment stretches over a period of time (mine lasted about a year), it is possible that there will be new developments regarding your particular type of cancer or the treatment for that cancer. Scientific studies are regularly being conducted on various types of cancers and the results of recently published studies may have an impact on your treatment and prognosis. If you have tied in to a support group connected with your type of cancer (especially an online group), that is an excellent resource for updates in the field concerning your condition and treatment. Check occasionally to see if anything has been published or if new treatments have received attention that you will want to discuss with your doctor. Although most good oncologists endeavor to keep up on all of the latest developments, do not assume that your doctor will have already heard about and considered the new sources. He may not have.[33]

Keeping informed also entails staying up to date on, and keeping your finger on the pulse of, what is going on with the people around you. Many times people want to shield a sick person from news or developments that may be unpleasant. But finding something out long after the fact, or finding out that information you would want to have known has been withheld from you, may only serve to aggravate you and increase your stress which, as discussed in chapters 1, 2 and 3, is detrimental to your recovery.

If your children are acting out or their grades are being affected by what you are going through, you will want to be aware of that. If your spouse is feeling depressed and worrying

---

33 The American Society of Clinical Oncology provides access to patients and their caregivers to articles published in the Journal of Clinical Oncology and the Journal of Oncology Practice. These journals can be a valuable resource in helping patients keep up to date on developments in cancer treatment. Information about gaining access to these journals can be found at www.cancer.net.

about your survival, you will want to reiterate to him how much you love him and how important his support has been to your progress. You may be able to share with him how you are progressing and reassure him. Let the people around you know if you want to be told about certain issues that come up outside of your own treatment. You can set the parameters of information you want to get. If there are topics you do *not* want to hear about (politics, in-laws, bills, etc.), be specific in telling those around you what you want to hear about and what you do not.

In addition, keeping yourself informed both about your condition and treatment, and how the other aspects of your life are being affected by your condition and treatment, can make you feel more in control of your situation. Feeling "in control" can help alleviate some of the stress that stems from a feeling of "helplessness" that may at times invade your thoughts.

Keep moving forward, and be QUICK about it.

CHAPTER 6

DEALING WITH CHEMOTHERAPY

"I make this look good."
Will Smith, *Men in Black*

Hearing that you will have to undergo chemotherapy can have daunting effects. Even people who have never dealt with it firsthand have some knowledge as to how onerous the treatments can be. They may have seen television shows or movies showing people undergoing chemotherapy. Perhaps they have had friends or relatives who have had to endure it. They know that it makes you lose your hair, feel nauseated and generally feel lousy. As a result, the prospect of going through chemotherapy can cause justified anxiety and stress.

The reality that I would have to go through chemotherapy is something that caused me a great deal of concern. My first treatment was to take place a few days after I entered the hospital and, as the day I would begin treatment crept closer, my trepidation rose. I found it difficult to turn my thoughts away from what chemotherapy would be like. What would happen to me? Would the treatment make me violently ill? Would I be throwing up all day? Would I be able to eat at all? Would I lose all of my hair and, if so, how soon would that happen? How would I look bald and possibly emaciated from the side effects of chemotherapy?

Truthfully, chemotherapy *is* onerous. While you may be one of the lucky ones who sail through it with little or no ill effects, for many people it makes them wonder whether the treatment is worse than the disease. The thing that helped me get through the "downs" of chemotherapy was to take my eyes off the *price* and keep them on the *prize*. If, like me, you can keep in mind the many things you have to live for, and the ultimate goal of chemotherapy, you will see chemotherapy for what it is: a small investment for a large return.

No Hair Up There (or Down There)

One common side effect of chemotherapy is hair loss. This effect, particularly for women, can be devastating. Being bald will make you look very, very different. Your appearance in the mirror will shock you, and your baldness will announce your cancer to those who know you when they come to see you or when you resume your life routines. It will remind you every day what you are going through, and chemotherapy is the culprit there.

Whereas, for men, baldness is generally accepted (and even represents a style choice for many men), the loss of hair often subconsciously affects a man's feelings about his virility (the decreased sex drive that can come with the fatigue and other effects of chemotherapy does not help). For women the issue is even more profound. Baldness in women simply is not accepted in most Western societies. Women often associate their hair with their beauty, and a woman's hair is something that men often note as a source of attraction. One need only view Botticelli's *Birth of Venus* to understand that long, flowing hair has long been a symbol of femininity. The loss of hair, therefore, particularly when that loss is sudden, can severely affect a cancer patient's self-image. Indeed, one of the first questions I asked the chemotherapy nurse assigned to me was, "Does everybody lose their hair?" I hoped I might be spared this effect (I am very vain, after all), but I was not.

Hair loss can progress differently for different patients, depending on the type of chemotherapeutic drugs being used, the dose administered and your nutrition. Your hair may fall out suddenly or in clumps. It may be lost gradually over a period of several days or weeks. You may lose it predominantly from your head or all over your body (including your eyelashes and eyebrows, chest hair and pubic hair). With newer, targeted methods of administering chemotherapy, however, hair loss may be minimal. There are different approaches to chemotherapy-induced baldness and you have the power to choose which approach to take.

You can choose to try to delay your hair loss as much as possible. There may simply be a limited amount you can do in this regard, but some things you can do to protect your hair for as long as possible (as well as your scalp, which may become sensitive) include: (i) avoiding harsh shampoos; (ii) brushing your hair minimally and with a soft brush, with spaced bristles; and (iii) letting your hair dry naturally, without using a blow dryer, and avoiding other heat sources like straighteners or heated rollers. If you decide to wear a wig during your bald period, get fitted for one before you begin treatment, if possible. That way, your wig can be matched to your natural hair color and will be available as soon as you need it. If you have long hair, you may be able to cut it before chemotherapy starts and fashion a wig from your own hair. Cutting your hair short will also have the effect of minimizing the appearance of thinning hair. If you cannot afford a wig, certain cancer organizations, including the American Cancer Society (www.cancer.org), have wig banks you can utilize.

You can embrace your new look. Not long after I began my

chemotherapy, I noticed that some strands of hair had begun to fall out and I mentioned this to my wife, Ceci. Looking at my still-full head of hair, she said, "No, it's not," and ran her hand innocently through it. When she looked down she realized that she was holding a handful of my hair. Almost disbelieving, she ran her hand through my hair again and came out with another handful. "Okay, enough," I said, initially repulsed by the sight of her easily removing clumps of my hair. The next day, however, upon further reflection, I decided that I had no desire to see more of it gone or sitting on my pillow each day. Instead, I used the clipper on my electric razor to shave my head, and asked my father to help shave the back of my head where I could not see what I was doing. I then paraded around the hospital ward paraphrasing Will Smith's character in *Men in Black*: "I make this look *good.*"

That approach helped both me and those around me deal with my new look in one fell swoop and adjust to it more quickly. When my daughters saw me later that evening on the videophone, they looked puzzled. Who was this bald guy who sounded like their father but did not look like him? When my elder daughter, Daniella, realized it was me she asked, "Abba, what happened to your hair?" Holding a bunch of her hair in her hands and lifting it up, she said, "You need hair, like me."

During my subsequent year of treatment, in between chemotherapy sessions, I continued to shave my head so that my children would not be confused by my constantly changing appearance as my hair grew back and then fell out again. I did, however, grow a goatee, which kind of gave me a tough look. In fact, sometime later, friends of ours told us that when they first moved in to our neighborhood (while I was donning this look), they did not realize I had cancer. The wife told her husband, who sports a deliberately shaved head and constantly changing permutations of facial hair, that he would "probably like that biker guy" (me). Cancer had actually given me the opportunity to look cool.

You can also be creative and have fun with how you cover your head if you choose to do so. You can choose the cap of your favorite sports team (cancer may even help you score an autographed hat from a favorite player if you write to the team). I have seen cancer patients wearing rainbow afros. I bought an Elmer Fudd–style hunting cap, complete with fold-down earflaps, to keep my head warm (you will notice how cold it is when you have no hair). When the son of friends of ours was diagnosed with cancer after I had gone through my treatment, I immediately ordered for him a set of "do-rags," complete with skulls, pirate insignias and motorcycle emblems, and encouraged him to look like a badass, instead of just the kid with cancer and a baseball hat (he loved them). A head covering will not only help limit the emotional effect of sudden baldness (on you and others), but will also protect your newly exposed scalp from the elements, especially sunlight. In this regard, you should also use sunblock on your scalp to protect yourself from sunburn (just make sure that you clear any particular sunblock you are considering using with your doctor before using it).

The bottom line is, although, like much of what happens with chemotherapy, the choices of *what* happens to you are limited, *how* you approach those consequences is *entirely* within your control. And bear in mind that your hair loss is only temporary. When your chemotherapy ends, your hair will most likely come back.

Oh, My Aching Stomach

Cancer patients tolerate the effects of chemotherapy differently. While some chemotherapy patients will experience no gastrointestinal side effects, however, most will experience at least some nausea, diarrhea, vomiting or constipation. This is because chemotherapy drugs attack rapidly dividing cells, like cancer cells, but also cells that line the stomach walls and digestive tract. Chemotherapy drugs also may stimulate responses in the brain that trigger nausea.

If you experience these symptoms, first and foremost inform your doctor or nurse. They will have access to medications that may help alleviate some of these effects, and there is no reason to suffer more than necessary in dealing with your cancer. Never be ashamed. Always remember that you are fighting the battle of your life, so the need to have your clothes or bedding changed, or even have someone stay with you, are small trifles. In addition, be proactive. If the anti-nausea or other drugs you are being given are not working for you, ask for something else. Thankfully, today there are several different types of such drugs that may be available to you and if one does not work, another may.

There are also other, nonmedicinal techniques that may help you deal with some of the gastrointestinal effects of chemotherapy. Eat smaller meals during the course of the day and avoid the impulse to eat quickly to "get it over with." To the contrary, eat slowly and chew thoroughly. This will make it easier for your body to tolerate the food you eat and digest it. Avoid heavy foods, particularly anything fried, fatty or very rich. Follow the general diet outline in chapter 14 and consult with a nutritionist to develop a nutrition plan that works for you. Stay well hydrated, as vomiting can raise the risk of dehydration, and avoid liquids that are either too hot or too cold. If you are experiencing nausea in general, avoid trying to eat your "favorite" foods during these times, to avoid a later negative association with those foods. If the smells of certain foods make you feel nauseated, ask whoever cooks in your house to refrain from cooking those items while you are going through your treatment.

Ask people who come to visit you or live with you to abstain from using items with strong fragrances, such as perfumes, colognes and deodorants, as strong smells can often trigger nausea. The same applies to using strong-smelling cleaning agents in your home. Arrange a time to be out when cleaning needs to be done in your home. Personally, the smell of the antibacterial hand soap in the hospital made me queasy. To this day, I still cannot bear it.

You can also try to manage your environment to calm yourself. Find a relaxing place to sit, breathe deeply to calm your muscles and nerves, listen to soft music and visualize yourself as a healthy person in a serene environment. For some people it is on the beach while the ocean waves roll in. For others it is on a mountain listening to the wind. For still others it is in their own home, watching their children play outside. It could be a place you have visited on a particularly good vacation. There are no rules. Whatever works to calm you down, focus on it and the waves of nausea will pass.

If your problem is more diarrhea, as it was for me, you must make sure to remain properly hydrated. Drink lots of the types of fluids referenced in chapter 14, and include natural, non-citrus fruit juices to replenish your electrolytes (just beware of juices that are very acidic and may exacerbate your stomach problems). Avoid liquids and foods that are either very hot or very cold. Use flushable baby wipes. They will save you from much of the discomfort that can accompany repeated trips to the bathroom.

Constipation is the other side of the chemotherapy coin. Some chemotherapy drugs or other drugs given to you to avoid nausea or diarrhea may cause constipation. Your doctor or nurse should be able to provide you with a laxative stimulant if constipation becomes a problem. You should also discuss with your doctor changes to your diet to include more high-fiber foods, some of which are listed in chapter 14. Again, proper hydration can help relieve constipation. Remember that, just as it is important to take in the nutrients your body needs to keep it strong and attack cancer cells, it is also vital that your body discharge wastes and toxins, and constipation, therefore, should not be approached cavalierly.

In addition, if you are spending more time in bed than usual and not getting the exercise you normally would, constipation may result. Emotional stress also can cause the body to stiffen and not release. Accordingly, you should try as much as you are able to move around and get some form of exercise. For myself, during my month-long initial hospital stay, I would repeatedly walk around the nurses' station with my IV pole just to get some exercise. We used to call it the IV Olympics. I would also use a Latin music tape my wife brought me to practice my (weak) dance moves in the waiting room, with my IV pole as my partner. Graceful, I was not, but at least I was moving, and you need to do so as well.

Tai chi is a wonderful, soft-style martial art and meditative exercise that can be helpful on many levels. Breathing is central to tai chi practice, and the movements involved are slow and fluid. They help stimulate circulation and gently raise your pulse. Tai chi movements also have lyrical names and the movements become, literally, poetry in motion. Moreover, several studies suggest that tai chi practice may be effective in helping to manage depression and anxiety and improve quality of life among patients with serious diseases, including cancer.[34] It may also improve immune function and increase the number of natural killer cells.[35] Basic tai chi instruction can be viewed on the Internet, can be practiced

34   See, e.g., W. C. Wang, et al., "The Effects of Tai Chi on Psychosocial Well-Being: A Systematic Review of Randomized Controlled Trials," *J Acupunct Meridian Stud.* (September 2009): 2(3):171–181; R. Jahnke, et al., "A Comprehensive Review of Health Benefits of Qigong and Tai Chi," *Am J Health Promot.* (July/August 2010): 24(6): e1–e25 at 11–12.

35   Ibid., 13, 16.

almost anywhere and is particularly enjoyable when practiced in a serene, natural setting (many tai chi groups practice in public parks). Millions of practitioners around the world can attest to its health-promoting effects. Having studied tai chi for several years in college, I was able to restart my practice when I was going through chemotherapy. Even in the hospital, although I could not perform some of the more difficult moves, there were many I could do, working in breathing techniques in the process. It also helped to center and relax me and thereby helped me avoid some of the combined effects of chemotherapy and lack of movement.

Is It Hot in Here, or Is That Just Me?

Depending on the type of chemotherapy drugs administered to you, your white blood cell counts may drop significantly. As a result, you may start running fevers as your body tries to deal with your cancer and your suppressed immunity. These fevers, especially if they spike (mine rose to over 104°), can be frightening. They can cause chills, rigor, sweating and a general feeling of malaise. They can exacerbate the other side effects of your treatment. For me, the sheer uncontrollability of the fevers I ran during chemotherapy and the fact that I could feel them coming on (I would begin to shake and feel cold) caused me a lot of anxiety. That anxiety was not entirely misplaced. Fever can be a sign of infection and, considering your immunosuppressed status, you should inform your doctor immediately if you start to run a fever during the course of your treatment. As a general rule of thumb, fever in an immunocompromised cancer patient should *always* be reported to his doctor and treated as an emergency until it is determined that no emergency exists.

Fever, however, is also your body's natural way of fighting disease. As Hippocrates said, "Give me a fever and I can cure any illness." Fever creates a condition in the body in which certain types of pathogens cannot survive and it accelerates the production of white blood cells. For this reason, although fevers during the course of your treatment can be uncomfortable and frightening, and may be a genuine cause for concern, they also are a sign that your body is doing what it is *supposed* to do. As discussed in chapter 15, this concept underlies hyperthermia treatments for cancer, inasmuch as cancer cells do not survive in elevated temperature environments. Ultimately, running fevers may simply be part of "sweating out" your disease.

Uh, What?

If you are going through chemotherapy, you may at some point experience a type of brain fog or inability to stay focused or concentrate. Sometimes this can occur following your chemotherapy sessions. This condition has come to be known as "chemo brain." It can take the form of not being able to remember names, dates or places, inability to perform work tasks or trouble collecting your thoughts. Radiation administered to the head for brain tumors may also cause this condition. The fatigue, sleep deprivation, disruption of your normal routines and stress attendant to having and being treated for cancer contribute to this unfocused feeling.

Experiencing chemo brain can be frightening and frustrating. But relax. You are not losing your mind. Most cases of chemo brain disappear a short time after treatment ends. Some of the techniques you can try to lessen its effects include:

- using a planner to keep track of your appointments and schedule your activities (make sure to keep it in a specific place so you don't wind up losing track of it);
- maintaining proper nutrition (see the basic dietary guidelines described in chapter 14);
- exercising; and

- doing activities to keep your brain sharp, such as playing games that require you to repeat and remember things ("I'm going on a picnic and I'm bringing …"), crossword puzzles and playing "memory" by placing playing cards facedown and trying to find the matches.

You should also let people know if you are experiencing chemo brain. As with other symptoms associated with your cancer or treatment, your doctors and nurses need to be kept aware of what you are experiencing. In addition, let the people around you know what is going on so they can help keep you organized and remain patient if you have momentary lapses. Let them know if there are particular things you are having trouble with so they can either help you with those things or perhaps take them off your hands.

Too Sexy for My Cancer?

Among the many things cancer and cancer treatments interfere with is your love life. Although while you are in the midst of being treated for cancer, sexual activity may be far from your mind—or even beyond your abilities—physical affection and sexual relations remain important to cancer patients (and their spouses or significant others). Indeed, on some levels, sexual intimacy may assume an even *more* important role when you are sick or undergoing treatment.

There are many reasons why battling cancer may interfere with your sex life, including, for example:

- physical discomfort attendant to surgery or in areas of the body that are sensitive due to radiation treatments or chemotherapy (in my own case, having an implanted mediport made certain types of movements uncomfortable, and my wife sometimes would inadvertently press against it, exacerbating the issue);
- fatigue flowing from the foregoing treatments or a hectic,

emotion-draining series of appointments and trips to the doctor or hospital;

- anxiety or stress over your diagnosis, which can interfere biologically with your ability to perform sexually or your desire to engage in sexual relations (this can be especially true for men treated for prostate or testicular cancer);
- body issues related to having had surgery (especially for women who have had surgery to treat breast cancer), baldness or weight loss; and
- hormonal changes stemming from your cancer treatment.

At the same time, the experience of enduring your cancer diagnosis and going through the rigors of treatment can increase both the need of a cancer patient to experience the love of his partner and the desire to have that love expressed through sexual relations. You may feel that you need to be reassured that you are still desirable and that your partner still sees you as attractive notwithstanding the changes you are going through.

A spouse or partner, on the other hand, may experience conflicting and sometimes colliding emotions. On the one hand, she may feel an increased desire to express her love for you in every way possible, including sexually. At the same time, however, she may be dealing with some of the same potential obstacles to resuming normal sexual relations as you, including her own concern and anxiety over your condition and the realities of physical changes you may be going through. They may worry about hurting you. They may also feel reluctant to press you for sex out of guilt or concern over your ability or desire to engage.

These effects of cancer and its remedies are common. In this area in particular, the key to maintaining the health of your relationship is to communicate with your partner. Let your husband or wife know what you are feeling, even if you do not feel physically or emotionally capable of engaging in sex. Ask him how *he* is feeling. After all, he may simply not understand that you are ready to resume that level of intimacy or how far you are capable of going. Sometimes, letting a person know that you want to be with them, but simply cannot, is enough to allay any concerns about rejection or how the other partner is feeling. It is perfectly fine to say, "Honey, I want so much to make love to you, but I just can't right now."

Nonetheless, if intimacy was an important part of your relationship before you were diagnosed with cancer, it will in all likelihood continue to be important after your diagnosis. Indeed, the vulnerability that cancer exposes in us can magnify the need and desire for such intimacy. There are also ways to approach sexual intimacy creatively or in ways that stop short of actual intercourse if that is too difficult. If physical discomfort is the issue, explore different positions to see if any of them make sex easier. Your partner may be able to use manual stimulation on you—or you on her—when intercourse is not feasible. The very act of satisfying your partner, even if it is not your usual way of doing so, can help rebuild your confidence in the strength of your physical relationship with her and relieve any sense on your part that you are being deficient in addressing those needs.

If you are otherwise feeling well enough to resume sexual relations but are experiencing a physical inability to perform, speak with your doctor about drugs or other treatments that may help. If the problem is more psychological, consider talking to a counselor or sex therapist to help you deal effectively with how your cancer and its ramifications are affecting your sex life in particular. While you or your spouse may feel some reluctance to opening up about this aspect of your cancer, the goal of reestablishing intimacy far outweighs the potential discomfort of talking about your feelings.

In addition, when sexual interaction is too taxing or is not possible, explore intimacy on another level. Affectionate relating that may have seemed "lesser" than sexual intercourse prior to cancer may take on another dimension when sex is not part of the equation. Foreplay may now become the main event. Such things as hand holding, hugging, kissing or even sitting close and experiencing together something you both enjoy (a movie, reading a book out loud, planning a vacation) can have gratifying results. In fact, they can reawaken in you the feelings of anticipation and eagerness for love that you experienced when you were first dating your spouse or partner. Take the time as well to write love letters to each other (you can even include racy details about the things you will do when you have defeated your cancer). You will be shoring up the foundations on which your sexual relationship was built in the first place.

When I was in the hospital and Ceci would come to visit me in the evenings (after my parents had gone to my house to babysit my children), she would sometimes just crawl into the hospital bed and lay next to me. It was a more intimate and important act than sexual intercourse ever could be. It reaffirmed to me the depth of our devotion to and need for each other, and that reaffirmation was one of my best treatments. As she told me during the course of my treatment: "When you have to say no to sex, say no to sex but yes to love."[36]

---

36   A related issue may be fertility if you and your spouse are planning to have more children. Some types of cancer treatments, including chemotherapy or radiation, can have reproductive effects, and you may want to speak to your doctor and a fertility specialist to make plans for storing eggs or sperm.

Listen to Your Body

Finally, even in the throes of cancer and chemotherapy, your body will still try to tell you when something is wrong. Listen to it. If you become feverish, break out in rashes or sores, experience dizziness, have physical pain, tingling or weakness or have other symptoms that just "don't feel right," tell your doctor and nurse. It may be that some of these and other symptoms are simply the by-products of your treatment, but some may not be, and it is vital that you listen closely to the messages your body sends and translate those messages to the people charged with your care. Again, now is no time to be bashful. Rest assured, the doctors and nurses caring for you have seen and heard it all, and they will not think ill of you for asking questions or expressing your fears or concerns.

CHAPTER 7

DEALING WITH RADIATION

"Mozart's music is like an X-ray of your soul
—it shows what is there, and what isn't."

Isaac Stern

Many people diagnosed with cancer will undergo radiation therapy (or "radiotherapy") as part of their treatment. Like chemotherapy, the prospect of going through radiation treatments can be frightening. The very thought of being "irradiated" conjures up scary thoughts about what the radiation will do to our bodies, especially as many of us have come to understand that exposure to excessive radiation may actually *cause* adverse health effects, including, perhaps, certain types of cancers. As such, you may have concerns that radiation treatments might cause some harm as well as good.

Radiation also can have some significant side effects, which may be worrying you. Some of those effects, such as nausea and other digestive problems, hair loss (which, while generally not as extensive with radiation as it is with chemotherapy, can occur in and around the areas being treated and may, in fact, be longer lasting or even permanent in those areas), as well as reproductive effects, are similar to what chemotherapy patients may experience. (Many of the recommendations contained in chapter 6 for dealing with those side effects during chemotherapy also are useful in dealing with them during radiation treatment.) The type and extent of radiation side effects depend largely on the dose administered and the areas of the body that are treated. Although these potential side effects may seem daunting, bear in mind that radiation therapy used for cancer treatment is dosed and monitored carefully and will be tailored to your specific type and stage of cancer. Moreover, like chemotherapy, radiation therapy has evolved and become more sophisticated over the years, such that several treatment and delivery options exist that may lessen these side effects, and techniques and medications exist that may help alleviate them.

Generally speaking, radiation therapy uses high-energy X-rays, electron beams or radioactive isotopes to target and kill cancer cells while minimizing the damage to healthy tissues surrounding those cancer cells. While the most common method of administering radiotherapy is externally, where radiation is directed at a specific area of the body in which a tumor is located, other means may include intravenous delivery or injection of radioactive solutions, or the implantation of radioactive seeds directly into a tumor.

Your therapy may involve a combination of these treatment methods. Ultimately, the goal is to deliver the maximum effective dose of radiation to a tumor and cancerous cells while limiting collateral damage to healthy tissue. This is one of the reasons why a regimen of radiotherapy often is spread out incrementally over multiple treatments. Which approach is right for you may depend on such factors as the location of your cancer and the possibility and types of side effects from a particular approach. As with other cancer treatments, therefore, you should discuss your options in detail with your oncologist, following the recommendations made elsewhere in this book regarding seeking out second opinions and other sources of information so that you can make an informed decision as to which treatment is best for you.

Getting Skinned

One of the most common side effects of radiation therapy (particularly external radiotherapy) is skin irritation, especially around the treated area. You may experience effects not unlike a bad sunburn, including dry skin, blistering or reddening, itchiness and peeling. It is important that you inform your oncologist or nurse if you start to experience these effects, as they may increase the chances of infection.

If you do experience these skin effects, be extra careful in how you treat the affected areas. For example, wear loose clothing made of natural fabrics (like cotton and linen) as opposed to man-made fabrics, which will not rub against sensitive areas as much as tight-fitting clothing and which provide protection against sun exposure to those areas. If your therapy is being applied to your head and neck area, wear a wide-brimmed, loose-fitting hat to protect your head and face from the sun. As hard as it may be, avoid rubbing or scratching the areas being treated as well. If the area needs to be covered with a bandage, avoid using types of bandages that have strong adhesives or surgical tape to attach bandages (paper tape often "sticks" less and hurts less when it is removed). If you live in a dry environment, or you are being treated during a dry season, use a humidifier in your home to lessen the dryness of your skin.

While ordinarily a hot bath or shower can be particularly soothing and help reduce stress, when you are going through radiotherapy you should avoid extremes of temperature and opt for warm showers instead of hot. Pat yourself dry with a soft towel or bath sheet instead of rubbing a towel against your body to avoid exacerbating any symptoms you may be experiencing. (For the same reasons, do not apply ice packs or heating pads to the affected areas.) Avoid soaps or shampoos with strong fragrances or deodorants (and if you are undergoing therapy, avoid washing off any markings that have been made on your body that determine where to deliver the radiation). Also, invest in good-quality sheets so that when you sleep, you lessen the amount of additional irritation to sensitive areas.

Although I never went through radiation therapy as part of my treatment, I know firsthand just how painful, disfiguring and downright miserable it can be to suffer these effects. During my episodes of Stevens-Johnson Syndrome, the skin in various parts of my body blistered and peeled off and the condition was so painful that even getting dressed was extremely uncomfortable. Many of the foregoing suggestions, however, helped me through those episodes, and may help you as well.

Most important, as with chemotherapy, there is no need to suffer in silence. Consult with your oncologist regarding creams or ointments that may alleviate some of the discomfort you are feeling. You may also receive recommendations from well-meaning friends to use certain creams or lotions. Some of these may be effective. Others, however, may have ingredients that may worsen any skin effects, so always consult with your oncologist before trying any remedies.

The Big Gulp

Radiotherapy applied to certain areas of the body, particularly the head and neck, can affect your throat and mouth, sometimes causing the lining of your throat to become inflamed or causing mouth ulcers, as well dry mouth. These side effects can make it hard to chew and swallow food. Radiation applied to the abdominal area can make you feel nauseated, vomit or cause diarrhea or abdominal discomfort. These effects in your mouth, throat and digestive tract can make eating unattractive or, in fact, simply uncomfortable. If you experience these effects, try eating foods that are softer and easier to swallow. Soups, vegetable juices, mashed sweet potatoes, pureed vegetables, oatmeal and eggs are some good choices. Also, cut your food into small pieces and chew thoroughly to make it easier to swallow.

In addition, avoid foods that are particularly acidic (like citrus and coffee), alcohol, spicy food and foods that are fried, salty, crunchy or sharp (like hard cereals and chips). If your mouth is very sensitive, use a straw to drink to direct liquids to parts of your mouth that may be less irritated. Avoid very hot or very cold foods and drinks. Eat smaller meals to lessen the amount of irritation you experience from eating or digestive issues. Blending, pureeing or juicing your food may help you get the nutrition you need simply by making it easier to swallow your food and keep it down. If necessary, consider using nutritional supplement drinks like Ensure to make sure you are getting the nutrients and calories you need. Use the techniques discussed in chapter 6 to help lessen any nausea you may feel and to help you deal with diarrhea or other digestive issues.

As with chemotherapy, your lack of desire to eat may lead you to avoid eating and drinking properly. As discussed in chapter 14, however, proper nutrition and hydration are critical to fighting your cancer, having the strength to deal with your treatments and carrying on with your other life activities as much as possible. The dietary suggestions in that chapter may help guide you in getting proper nutrition notwithstanding the side effects of your treatment, and you should also consult a cancer nutritionist to get additional helpful suggestions. Further, discuss with your doctor methods to lessen your discomfort, as there may be antacids and painkillers (like a lidocaine-based mouth rinse, which I used during my SJS episodes, or gels to coat your throat) that can alleviate your pain at least temporarily and thereby allow you to eat and drink properly.

You should also make sure to practice good oral hygiene even if your mouth is sore. Check your mouth on a daily basis to spot any problems when they start, so that they can be reported to your oncologist and treated as soon as possible and hopefully reduced. Drink plenty of water during the day to keep your mouth tissues moist. Make sure to brush your teeth regularly but use gentle toothpaste, like Biotene, to avoid irritating your mouth further. Do not use alcohol-based mouthwashes. Continue to floss your teeth but do so very gently to avoid cutting or irritating your gums. You are going to be smiling and laughing a lot when you are finished with your treatments, so do whatever you can to make that smile as good as it can be.

I also dealt with the effects of severe mouth and throat ulcers during my bouts with Stevens-Johnson Syndrome. The insides of my mouth and throat, as well as the surface of my lips and tongue, literally blistered and came off, making eating and drinking incredibly painful. There were times when I could only consume liquids and, even then, only by using a straw and directing what I was drinking to specific parts of my mouth. Even when those episodes were at their worst, however, employing some of the approaches described above helped me get the nutrition I needed, and they may help you too.

Radiation Down Under

Radiotherapy applied to the pelvic area or prostate brings its own set of potential side effects. These can include bladder-related issues, such as difficulty urinating or painful urination, incontinence, a feeling that you need to urinate often and cramps. Most of these effects resolve within a few weeks of finishing your treatments. If you experience these effects, make sure to hydrate properly and avoid foods and liquids (coffee, alcohol and spicy foods) that may exacerbate discomfort while urinating. Your oncologist or a therapist may also be able to recommend certain exercises to help you control your bladder.

Treatment to these areas of your body—and going through cancer and its treatments generally—also may have sexual or reproductive effects. Interest in sex may decrease, sexual intercourse may be painful or, for men, erectile dysfunction can occur. Review the discussion of sexual intimacy during chemotherapy in chapter 6 to address how to interact with your partner if sexual arousal or intercourse become difficult during your radiation therapy. They will help you achieve and experience intimacy—even if that intimacy stops short of actual sexual intercourse—during your treatment.

Because fertility also may be affected as a result of your treatment, discuss your options (such as storing sperm or eggs) with a reproductive specialist before you begin your treatment. Not knowing what the long-term effects of my chemotherapy would be, I chose this route myself and it gave me great peace of mind during my treatment to know that I had kept my options open by doing so. For women who are going to be receiving radiation in their pelvic area, it may be possible to have your ovaries actually moved out of the field of radiation through a relatively simple laparoscopic procedure, thereby preserving fertility. Discuss this option with your oncologist before you begin radiation treatments to see if you are a candidate for such a procedure.

Thankfully, we live in a world where for many people pregnancy can be achieved even where reproductive difficulties exist. If you are hoping to have children following your treatment, do not leave these stones unturned. As discussed in many places in this book, there is life—*great life*—after cancer, and you should endeavor to take advantage of every possible aspect of it.

CHAPTER 8

PROTECTING YOURSELF
DURING YOUR TREATMENT

"Be careful about reading health books.
You may die of a misprint."
Mark Twain

If you are hospitalized during your treatment, or even if you are being treated as an outpatient and convalescing at home, many of your friends and relatives will want to come see you. Many cancer patients look forward to such visits. The support and humor of friends and loved ones can be an enormous source of encouragement and can lift your spirits tremendously, which is a vital element in the ultimate success of your treatment. It is of utmost importance, however, that you be honest with yourself and others in terms of whether such visits are a good idea.

No Such Thing as a Little Sniffle

If you are undergoing chemotherapy or radiation, or are recovering from surgery, the fact is that your body's defenses may be down. You may be very drained physically. Your immune system may be particularly compromised. As a result, you will be very susceptible to contracting additional illnesses from other, well-meaning, people. People come into contact with the germs and diseases of others every day in their workplaces, schools and even in public places like the supermarket or the subway. This is especially so during winter months, when colds and flu are common. Children, who are constantly exposed to other children in school who are sick during winter months, are a particular risk for exposure. Someone else's little sniffle, which might not cause you any concern when you are well, is a serious cause for concern when you are immunocompromised by your cancer or your treatment.

As much as you may look forward to visits from friends and relatives, you may need to avoid them. If your body is telling you that you are exhausted, or your symptoms indicate that you are immunocompromised (if, for example, you are running a fever or are feeling particularly weak), you need to be firm with yourself and others and limit your exposure to other people. This can be very hard, especially if those other people are your children or close friends.

In my own case, this was very difficult. My children were very young and not being able to see them for the month of my hospitalization was, without exception, the most depressing part of having cancer. Luckily, the hospital provided me with a videophone that I could use to at least see them and let them see and talk to me every day. Now, this option is even greater, as Internet-available programs, such as Skype and Oovoo, allow you to actually see and talk to people without being in the same room (or even the same city, state or country) as them. Take advantage of modern technology. It will allow you to get the love and support you need from people without endangering yourself.

Do not worry about offending people who want to visit you. Be honest with them. Tell them that as much as you appreciate their kindness and would love to have them come visit you, you need to avoid potential exposure to illnesses during your treatment and convalescence, or explain that you are simply too tired to have visitors. They will understand, and delaying your visits with them for the time being is another small investment in hardship that will pay bigger dividends when you are feeling better and are able to spend time with your loved ones without risking your health.

When people do come to see you, do not be afraid to make them take precautions. If you are particularly at risk, ask them to don surgical masks or gloves (or use them yourself). The hospital or your doctor will in all likelihood make these available to you. Ask them to wash their hands when they come into your home or hospital room, or keep a container of antiseptic/antibacterial hand sanitizer available and ask them to use it when they come in. No guest who came to visit me ever registered an iota of annoyance when I told them to wash their hands before they came into my hospital room. Moreover, as much as you may need to have their hugs and kisses, be strong and do without them. Blow kisses and tell them that you love them, and explain that you simply cannot hug and kiss right now, but that you will take those hugs and kisses with interest as soon as it is safe to do so.

You also need to be cautious in the hospital itself. In some respects, the hospital is the *worst* place to be when you are sick, simply because you are surrounded by sick people. If you are able to have a private room, that will help insulate you to some extent. While there is certainly some comfort to be gained from interacting with other patients (your comrades in arms) and encouraging each other, be wary of exposing yourself or them to potential complications. In addition, although most hospitals strive to make sure that their rooms are cleaned thoroughly between patients (and while patients are in them), certain areas may escape a thorough cleaning. These may include items and areas most patients will be in contact with, such as telephones, television remotes, doorknobs, call buttons, bedrails and guest chairs. Cleaning staff in even the best hospitals may miss these areas, which can accumulate germs and bacteria from prior users or even guests who come to visit a patient. As such, one way you may avoid exposures from these items which may complicate or interfere with your recovery, especially if you are immunocompromised, is by using Clorox wipes (or a similar bleach-based cleaner) to wipe down these items before you use or come into contact with them. Using such precautions truly can bring home the old adage that "an ounce of prevention is worth a pound of cure."

To Sleep, Perchance to Dream (About Being Healthy)

In addition, your treatments may leave you exhausted. Rest is an essential element in your recovery. Indeed, as Thomas Dekker wrote back in 1609, "Sleepe is the golden chain that ties health and our bodies together." Thus, although again the scientific evidence is mixed, there is evidence to suggest that getting proper sleep may be associated with your body's ability to defeat your cancer.

For example, a 2003 study undertaken at Stanford University indicates that sleep deprivation inhibits the body's production of melatonin, which is an antioxidant that helps eliminate free radicals. Less melatonin linked to sleep deprivation may, therefore, lead to a situation where a cell's DNA is more susceptible to cancer-causing mutations.[37] Further, melatonin slows a woman's production of estrogen, a hormone that some studies have linked to cancerous cell reproduction in ovarian and breast cancers.[38]

---

37 See S. Sephton and D. Spiegel, "Circadian Disruption in Cancer: A Neuroendocrine-Immune Pathway from Stress to Disease?" *Brain, Behavior and Immunity* (2003): 17: 321–328 at p. 323 (the "Sephton study").

38 Ibid. The authors reference other studies in which breast cancer incidence was determined to be higher in women who worked night shifts, which may have altered their melatonin and cortisol production.

Animal and human studies suggest that insufficient sleep may aid in cancer progression.[39] The Sephton study also indicated that disrupted sleep patterns may suppress immune-based cancer defenses and reduce the efficacy of chemotherapy drugs.[40] Another study demonstrated that interference with the "circadian clock"—the internal clock in our bodies that tells us when to go to sleep and when to wake up—of test animals led to significant acceleration in tumor growth.[41] It should be noted, however, that the results of animal studies are difficult to extrapolate to human experience. Different species react differently to stimuli, treatments and diseases and, therefore, just because something happens in a mouse does not mean that it necessarily will happen in a person.

Thus, proper sleep—and the opportunity for the body to repair itself during sleep hours—is potentially an important tool to help you heal. Even putting aside whether insufficient sleep can or cannot affect cancer initiation and progression, getting enough rest can help improve your mood, reduce your stress and boost your energy level, all vital components in your quest to get well.

Unfortunately, for many of us, it is also one of the things that is hardest to come by. There are a number of things that can interfere with sleep when you have cancer and are being treated for it. First, the physical effects themselves, be they physical pain caused by a cancerous growth or the discomfort attendant to cancer surgery, can make it difficult to get comfortable. The medi-port I had and being connected to an IV all the time made it virtually impossible to sleep in any position other than flat on my back, which I generally had not done previously.

---

39   Ibid., 324–325, 327.

40   Ibid., 326–327.

41   E. Filipski, et al., "Disruption of Circadian Coordination and Malignant Growth," *Cancer Causes Control* (May 2006): 17(4): 509–514.

Side effects of conventional cancer treatments like chemotherapy and radiation also can interfere with sleep patterns. Being in a hospital, where there is constant noise outside your room and people come in to check on you every four hours, effectively precludes a normal sleep pattern. Also, the stress and anxiety that can be part of having and being treated for cancer can keep you up at all hours of the night.

Indeed, my first night in the hospital was the day after my diagnosis. The hospital felt strange and alien. I was dealing with the emotions of my diagnosis and prognosis. I missed my family already. Needless to say, that first night was not very restful. The next morning I was dozing in bed when a doctor who was doing rounds came into my room with a group of young doctors in tow observing him. Upon seeing me nodding off in bed, he said, rather curtly, "It's eight o'clock already," indicating that he clearly felt that I should be up and alert for him. His attitude made me angry. It was, after all, less than forty-eight hours after I was diagnosed, and I was confused as to exactly what cancer patient etiquette he thought I was violating.

"Did someone come to your house last night and wake you up every four hours to check your vitals?" I asked him.

"No," he said.

"Then leave me alone," I shot back. If I could not sleep, at least I would not be hassled about it.

This is an aspect of cancer that can be dealt with, however. The numerous stress-reduction techniques described elsewhere in this book should be utilized as a frontline approach to cancer-related sleep problems. You may find that using them helps you recover your ability to sleep normally. Develop a sleep routine and stick to it. Try to go to sleep at the same time each night and get up the same time each morning. In addition, spend as much of your awake time as possible out of bed, so that your bed will be associated only with sleeping (and, hopefully, intimacy), as opposed to waiting around for, thinking about and receiving your treatments. If there are specific stress-reduction techniques that are particularly helpful to you in reducing your stress and enhancing your relaxation, work them into your sleep routine. As I settled into my hospital "sleep routine" over the ensuing weeks, which included "shutting down" certain stimuli (for example, by turning off the television and the ringer on the phone, lowering the lights and closing my hospital room door to shut out some of the hallway noise), I found that it was easier to get to sleep.

In the alternative, there are various sleep aids that you can use to help restore your sleep patterns. Among the natural supplements that have been associated with improving sleep are melatonin and valerian root. Melatonin has been shown to affect both how quickly people fall asleep and the duration of their sleep.[42] Although the scientific evidence on the efficacy of valerian root is not dispositive of whether it is an effective sleep aid, its use for such purposes stretches back centuries. In fact, as far back as the second century, the Greek physician, surgeon and philosopher Galen of Pergamon prescribed valerian root to treat insomnia. It is available in several forms, including tea, drops to add to a beverage or supplement pills.[43]

Conventional sleeping pills may also be of assistance in helping you get the sleep you need, and an appropriate one for you can be discussed with your doctor. *As with any course of treatment or supplements you may consider using, discuss their use with your doctor first to make sure there are*

---

42 *Complete Guide to Complementary & Alternative Cancer Therapies,* 797.

43 For a discussion of the various studies that have been done on the use of valerian root as a sleep aid, *see* the National Institute of Health's Dietary Supplement Fact Sheet for Valerian, available at http://ods. od.nih.gov/factsheets/valerian.

no contraindications either for your condition or the other medicines you are taking. In addition, if you are hospitalized, your doctor may be amenable to modifying your monitoring schedule (for example, by reducing the frequency of vital sign and temperature checks during the night or employing an electronic monitor during sleep hours) to limit interruptions that may prevent you from getting the rest you need.

Whether in the hospital or at home, a good rule to follow is, again, simply to listen to your body. It will tell you when you are too sick or tired for certain activities or visits from friends or relatives. Many cancer patients feel a burst of desire to forcibly make themselves well. You may feel an increased need to exercise or "get back in the game" in terms of work or other activities. You may feel compelled to show yourself or others that your cancer is not going to beat you, and that is laudable. It can also be detrimental, however, if in fact your body is not as prepared as your mind to do such things. When you are tired, rest. When you are feeling sick or run-down, dial back your activities. As you begin to feel stronger, work in additional activities and responsibilities incrementally and build up your strength gradually. The last thing you want to do is overstress your system into breaking down. Take the time to let your body catch up and repair itself. It will let you know when it is time to resume your full schedule.

PART II

A Little Thing That Makes a Big Difference

The Positive Cancer Attitude

CHAPTER 9

LIVE THE CLICHÉ: LAUGHTER AND JOY

*"Resolve to keep happy and your joy and you shall
form an invincible host against difficulties."*

Helen Keller

You have probably heard the old adage that "laughter is the
best medicine." Indeed, the belief that "a merry heart is like
a good medicine"[44] has been expressed for millennia. There are,
in fact, studies that lend support to this long-held belief and
the health-promoting effects of real, sincere laughter.

For example, a British study analyzed the effects of laughter
on pain reduction. Study volunteers watched episodes of
popular television or stage comedies whereas other volunteers
watched stage dramas, golf or wildlife programs. Pain was
applied in the form of a frozen wine cooler sleeve slipped onto
the participants' arms. The study demonstrated that, while
fifteen minutes of genuine, relaxed, unforced laughter from
watching comedies increased pain tolerance by 10 percent,
watching the non-comedy programs had no effect on pain
reduction. This decrease in pain was related to the release of
endorphins—chemicals that dull signals of physical pain and

---

44 Proverbs 17:22.

psychological stress transmitted between neurons—triggered by the physical effort (the muscular exertions) involved in laughter.[45]

Additional studies conducted by Drs. Lee Berk and Stanley Tan of Loma Linda University Medical Center in California indicate that laughter, among other things: (i) helps relieve pain; (ii) improves mood; (iii) lowers blood pressure; (iv) reduces stress hormones; (v) increases muscle relaxation; (vi) decreases anxiety and fear; and (vii) boosts the immune system. They also have demonstrated that laughter raises the levels of infection-fighting T cells, disease-fighting proteins called gamma interferon and B cells, which produce disease-destroying antibodies. Our emotions, particularly positive emotions, also may affect our immune systems through the release of neurotransmitters such as serotonin, dopamine and norepinephrine, which are injected into the bloodstream and act on white blood cells.[46]

It Only Hurts Less When I Laugh

The very idea of being joyful and laughing heartily when you have cancer or are undergoing the rigorous treatments involved in fighting your cancer can seem alien. There may simply seem to be nothing funny at all in your situation. You must endeavor, however, to try to see and seek humor wherever you can, as it may help you heal. After all, when you

---

45 See R. I. M. Dunbar, et al., "Social Laughter is Correlated with an Elevated Pain Threshold," *Proc. R. Soc. B* (August 2011), 5.

46 Ibid. Similarly, a study examined the immune response of subjects watching videos describing the work of Mother Teresa whereas other subjects watched footage of the Vietnam War. Subjects watching the Mother Teresa videos showed a more positive immune response than the other subjects. See A. Chatham, MPhil, MTh, MSW, "Our Emotions Can Create White Blood Cells," *Healing Our World*, vol. 31, no. 4 (Hippocrates Health Institute, 2011).

really think about it, there is virtually nothing in the realm of comedy that is "off limits." Often times the funniest comedic bits are dark, focusing on things like marital distress ("Take my wife, please." —Henny Youngman), racial tensions ("None of you would change places with me. And I'm rich! That's how good it is to be white." —Chris Rock), drug abuse ("To say that you do just a little cocaine is like saying you're swimming with just a small shark." —Robin Williams). Cancer is no different. Find the funny things and laugh at them.

People will ask you what they can do to help you, and they will *desperately* want to do so. Tell them to tell you the funniest jokes they know. Ask them to send you comedy DVDs or direct you to the funniest video clips they have seen. Have them share amusing stories with you. Not only will it make you feel better, but it will make *them* feel better to see you in good spirits and participate in your recovery. It will help lessen the feeling of helplessness your loved ones feel in watching you go through your ordeal.

Although I had not yet seen many of the studies demonstrating the link between laughter/joy and healing, I was very resolved when I was hospitalized and going through chemotherapy to try as much as possible to approach everything with humor. I knew that it would make things easier for my wife, children, parents and friends, and I sought out ways to make things humorous. Some of you may have used a service called "Moviephone" when searching for a movie to see. It includes a recording directing you to choose from a list of current movies or say the name of the movie you want to see to hear which theatres in your area are playing it. I used that message as a model for my hospital answering machine and composed the following message for incoming calls:

Hello, and welcome to cancer phone. If you know the name of the cancer you would like to hear about, press 1. To choose from a list of current cancers, press 2.

To find out which cancers are prevalent in your area, press 3. If you want to leave a message for Howard, please start speaking after the tone. Have a great day, and remember, bald is beautiful.

A few of my friends were put off by the message. Others were confused, believing at first that they had reached a hospital service in error. But most people appreciated the humor, telling me later that my message had helped them relax and get past the anxiety of not knowing what to say to me. It broke the ice and remains something that my friends remember and laugh at to this day.

Early in my hospital stay, the reproductive specialist came to see me. He advised me that, if I was hoping to have more children after my treatment, I should consider storing some sperm. The nurse politely offered to put a note on my door advising that I not be disturbed while I did what I had to to give the doctor a specimen for storage. "What's wrong," I asked, "don't you have a 'Do Not Enter: Patient Masturbating' sign out there?" She broke up laughing, and I proceeded to do what was necessary.

On another occasion, a young, female doctor was performing a bone marrow biopsy on me. The procedure is done at the hip, but it requires that you be exposed pretty much from the waist down. She performed the procedure quickly and well, and when it was done she said that she was going to continue applying pressure to the incision to stop the bleeding. "Sure," I said, "you just want to keep your hands on my ass." She was a good sport.

During my consolidation chemotherapy treatments, I was required to have a bone marrow biopsy once a month. This is a very painful procedure (although done correctly, it does not take that long). On one occasion, I had the procedure performed only to have the doctor call me later in the day to tell me, with profuse apologies, that I would have to repeat the procedure the next day because he had failed to actually extract marrow. "Fine," I told him, "but first I'm going to do one on *you*."

On yet another occasion, I was in the hospital elevator on my way, again, to a bone marrow biopsy. Another patient asked me about the procedure, how much it hurt and whether the lidocaine injections given before the procedure helped alleviate some of the pain. "Actually, it's a pretty fast procedure so the doctor doesn't give me any lidocaine," I teased. "He just gives me a tongue depressor to bite down on." She was shocked and horrified, but I told her right away that, of course, I was kidding and that the procedure, while painful, was pretty quick. (In fact, for patients who simply cannot tolerate the procedure, they sometimes can be placed under sedation to avoid this discomfort.)

Humor, even if it is dark or self-deprecating, can bring you and others up when you otherwise would be down.

Brighten Up and Smile Right

Bringing up the spirit of your surroundings is also up to you. Many hospital rooms are drab and plain. They often lack an inspiring array of colors. The hospital may control what gets put on its own common walls, but when it comes to your space, *make it yours*. In your own home, you run the whole show. Whether at home or in the hospital, start with adding some color. Many studies have shown that colors have an impact on mood. For example, in a study conducted at Vrije Universiteit in Amsterdam, subjects reported feeling happier when surrounded by green and yellow colors. These colors suggest sunshine, warmer climates and natural surroundings. Blues, which remind us of the ocean or a clear sky, tend to have a calming effect. Several studies, including those by Nancy J. Stone, PhD, professor of psychology at Creighton University in Omaha, Nebraska, have found that people faced with difficult or stressful tasks felt calmer after they focused on something blue.[47]

Have someone bring you some colored balloons or bright flowers (if you are allowed to have them in your room), or ask your children or grandchildren to make colorful pictures for you. In addition, do not limit yourself to the same redundant, drab hospital gowns. If possible, use your own clothing and pajamas, or have someone get you new ones with good coloring. You can also find doctor's scrubs with bright designs and cartoon characters on them, and they are extremely comfortable.

When I first checked into the hospital, entering the room that would be my "home away from home" for an indeterminate amount of time made me feel sad and lonely. Much like a convict feels his incarceration most profoundly the first time a cell door clangs shut behind him, walking into my hospital room brought home with full force what I was facing. I began to get a lump in my throat and I fought back the desire to turn around and leave immediately, which, in any event, was not an option.

Instead, I tried to reassure my wife and myself that the room was not so bad. In fact, it was private, spacious, had a comfortable reclining guest chair, a closet, a large window and a private bathroom. It was like a "chemo condo." But it was still a hospital room, one in which I would be a "guest" for some time, so I endeavored to "own it" as much as possible. I put my things in the closet, including my own clothes and pajamas. I changed immediately into a set of doctor's scrubs (as this was before I lost my hair, if I had thrown a stethoscope around my neck it would have been hard to distinguish me from any nice Jewish doctor roaming the halls of the hospital).

---

47 See, e.g., A. Hoicowitz, et al., "How Color Affects Mood," at http://jrscience.wcp.muohio.edu/nsfall99/labpacketArticles/Final1.How-ColorAffectsMoo.html.

I placed the pictures of my children where I could see them and arranged my books and other personal items. I plugged in my laptop.

I also had my wife bring me my daughter's Pocahontas blanket. A lot of people commented on and laughed at it, but it brought a lot of life and color to my room, made *me* laugh, reminded me of my children and made me feel their presence, and made the bed I had to spend so much time in more appealing. It also made me feel warm in many ways when my feverish chills would come on. In essence, making the hospital room "my own" made it more comfortable and made the prospect of a long and difficult stay more palatable.

In addition to the beneficial effects of surrounding yourself with laughter and brightness and "owning" your situation, setting your mood and seeking out things that make you feel good is yet another way to reclaim the control over your life that cancer may have pilfered from you. Indeed, finding laughter and joy in the face of the challenges that cancer gives us is itself a form of courage. If you have hobbies that are not precluded by your condition, continue doing them. Play an instrument. Paint. Write poetry. Do yoga.

During the year of my treatment, I rediscovered my tai chi practice. I also learned how to really cook and bake. I got my mother-in-law's ceviche recipe and tried it out. It was not overly stressful on my system and it made me feel that I was contributing something on the home front, particularly for my wife, who put up with so much. Each night she would come home to a new aroma and even some Latin-American delicacies after a long day. For the person who brought me the most comfort, at least I could give her some Peruvian comfort food to bring back good memories of her country of origin. My culinary experiments even earned me a reputation in the neighborhood as a dessert specialist.

If you feel up to it, you can also continue to be involved in work. You can even participate in conference calls or videoconferences if you cannot attend physically. I actually participated in a conference call in the hospital, *during a bone marrow biopsy*. It generally took my mind off what was being done to me, although the conversation was interrupted with some strong exclamations. Continuing to be involved can produce an additional, positive emotion that will aid in getting you through your treatment and maybe even your healing process.

A kiss for good luck and good health from Daniella.

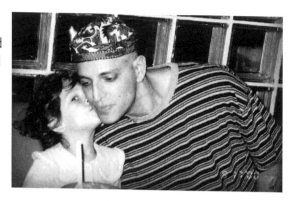

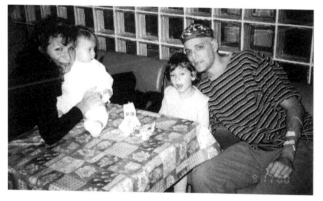

The best medicine: Ceci, Michal and Daniella visiting me toward the end of my hospital stay.

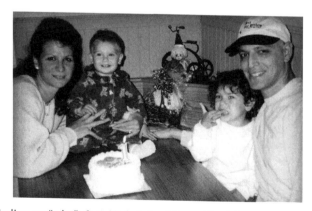

Finding my "why": Ceci, Michal, Daniella and I celebrating Michal's first birthday right after my discharge from the hospital.

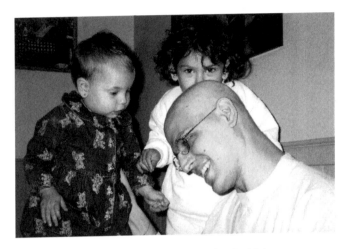

Michal and Daniella getting used to Daddy's new
look and feel on Michal's first birthday.

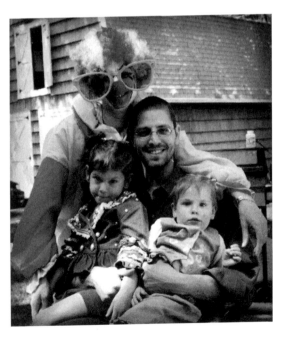

On the road back to health: Celebrating Daniella's fourth birthday and
clowning around with Ceci toward the end of my chemotherapy.

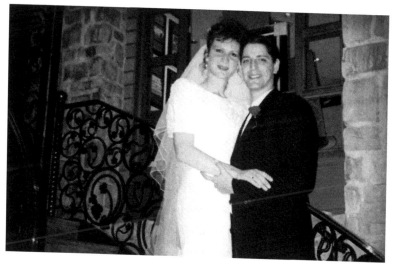

Renewing our vows in Las Vegas after the completion of my chemotherapy.

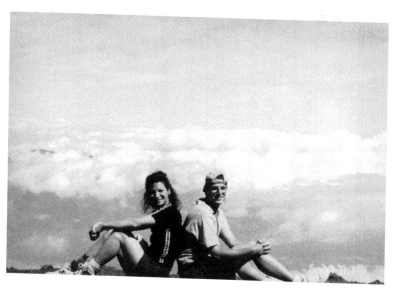

Reaching new heights: On the summit of Haleakala in Hawaii on our second honeymoon, following our renewal of vows in Las Vegas.

CHAPTER 10

BE NORMAL

"Nobody realizes that some people expend tremendous energy merely to be normal."
Albert Camus, *Notebook IV, Notebooks: 1942-1951*

When you have been diagnosed with cancer or are undergoing treatment for it, your life is anything but normal. Indeed, your entire sense of normalcy has probably been thrown into complete disarray. It is human nature to rely on routines. We attune our mental and physical clocks to those routines: getting up at a certain time in the morning, getting children ready and out for school, getting to and leaving work at set hours, going to the gym, moving between scheduled extracurricular activities and other things become interwoven with our psyches and how our bodies function. As much as we may complain about the hectic pace of our schedules, most of us, consciously or subconsciously, come to rely on having those routines. Being able to anticipate what our days will bring provides a certain sense of comfort and allays fears of the unknown.

That is why a disruption in our routines can be so traumatic. Beyond the immediate financial issues, the loss of a job is so disturbing in part because it disrupts our sense of normalcy. Instead of predictably having someplace to go every day, all of a sudden the day is left without direction or a sense of accomplishment. When children leave home to go to school or move into their own apartment, the sudden lack of someone else who relies on us, shares in our daily routines, engages us in conversation or simply makes noise around the house can be very discomforting and disorienting.

Cancer or other significant diseases can have the same effect. There are few things that can shake your core of normalcy as badly as being told that the one thing you have come to rely on more than anything—your life—could itself be taken from you long before you expected it to be. Moreover, all of a sudden, you may not be able to work (or may be able to work only part-time). Maybe you will not be able to help around the house, drive your car, carry heavy packages, perform sexually, toilet independently or even stay awake to participate in family activities. As much as we may sometimes complain about these chores, the *ability* to do them when we choose or have to is important to us, even when we are not thinking consciously about that ability. Losing that ability means losing some of your independence and, worse, becoming dependent on others to help you with basic tasks. These effects of cancer and cancer treatments can thereby have a detrimental, depressive effect on cancer patients. Those depressive effects, which also can trigger your stress response, need to be reduced as much as possible.

The answer is to be normal. In other words, do as many things as you can that are part of your normal routine. On the battlefield, soldiers are often directed to shave on a daily basis. Why? Because it reinforces a sense of normalcy under abnormal circumstances. It helps re-center the soldiers by reminding them of their routines under normal circumstances, and reduces their anxiety. Indeed, research has shown that people (and even animals) engage in ritualistic behaviors to induce a sense of calm in circumstances they perceive as being unpredictable or uncontrollable. Engaging in such rituals contributes to a general feeling of being in control and reduces stress.[48] Put simply, feeling normal as a result of doing normal things is good for you.

Even if you are not going to work, you can still get dressed every day. Do not sit around in your pajamas all day long. Even if you need to nap during the day, put on clothes in the morning that are easy to remove if you want to lie down for a while. Change your clothes daily as well. Do not put on the same clothes or pajamas on consecutive days. In fact, buy yourself some new clothing and intersperse them in your wardrobe to give yourself a fresh new look as you go through your treatment. Buy a few special things to wear at milestones in your treatment, such as when you complete a round of chemotherapy or radiation, or even more so for when you are told that you are cancer free. Even in the hospital, you can get dressed, and changing out of hospital garb and seeing yourself—and letting others see you—dressed and looking good can have substantial, beneficial emotional results.

When I went into the hospital to begin my treatment, I made a point of bringing with me a nice pair of pants and a couple of dress shirts for the Sabbath. I did not wind up wearing them every week I was there, but putting them on for even a little while made my situation feel less strange and reminded me that there was, indeed, life beyond the hospital walls.

Keep up your grooming habits as well. Provided your treatments do not prevent you from doing so (for example, because your skin is very sensitive or cutting yourself presents a dangerous situation), shave or put on makeup as you would on any other day. Brush and style your hair if you still have it

---

48   D. Eilam, et al., "Threat Detection: Behavioral Practices in Animals and Humans," *Neurosci Biobehav Rev.* (March 2011): 35(4): 999–1006.

(and if you don't, keep whatever head covering you use clean or have different ones for different days). These things will make you feel better about yourself and reassure those around you. If exercise is part of your normal routine, keep doing it. If your regular exercises are not possible, seek out other, less stressful exercises, including those discussed in chapters 1 and 6, and do them at the same time as you would do your regular routine. Even many of your social interactions—book clubs, card games and coffee klatches—can be available to you either in person or online if you cannot be there.

When I was first diagnosed, it was customary for different members of my synagogue to deliver the weekly Sabbath sermon, something I did several times. When one of the service organizers called to ask me how I was feeling, I told him, "I want to give the sermon this week." He thought I was kidding, but I meant it. I worked up a sermon dealing with people performing acts of kindness for others, and thanking my many friends for doing so for me and my family, and e-mailed it to my friend, who read it for me that weekend in synagogue.

As my strength began to return, I started to reclaim some of my work responsibilities. The oral chemotherapy I was on at that time gave me constant, brutal headaches and, even during the course of one of the largest toxic tort trials in American history, there were times when I had to discipline myself and tell the other team members that I was finished for the day. Yet being involved in these things made me feel more normal.

Investigate as well the possibility of having your treatments administered at home. While many cancer patients must be treated in a hospital setting, many medications can be administered by home care specialists, such as visiting nurse services, and some—including certain types of chemotherapy and antibiotic injections—can be given either by a family member or the patient himself. Arranging for these treatments to be given in your home can help you avoid time-consuming, tiresome and disrupting trips to the doctor's office or hospital. As such, they can help you maintain a more normal routine.

The challenges of chemotherapy instructed me as to the value of good, old, boring "normal." Indeed, to paraphrase William James, going through the abnormal is "the best way of understanding [and, I would add, appreciating] the normal."

CHAPTER 11

"WHEN IT'S DARK ENOUGH,
YOU CAN SEE THE STARS"

This quote, from Ralph Waldo Emerson, is an exhortation to recognize that, even at the darkest hour, there are points of light to guide us to where we need to go, cheer us and chase away the fear of the unknown. There will almost certainly be times during your cancer treatment when you will find yourself in a dark place; sad, depressed, frightened, angry. Maybe it will be at night when you are having trouble sleeping and you are worrying about how your treatment is going and whether you can get through it. Perhaps it will be at the end of visiting hours when you have said good-bye to your loved ones and are facing another night alone. Or maybe those dark times will come during a particularly rough chemotherapy session or if you have had a setback in your progress.

I remember an especially difficult evening, after my wife had left to go home to attend to the children and I had had my daily phone call with them and wished them a good night. I sat on my bed, looking out the window at an outside life I had not been able to experience in weeks, and felt the heaviness coming into my soul. I felt the weight of sadness that wells up right before a particularly heavy crying session.

One of the night-shift nurses who had come in to check on me saw my expression and asked if I was all right. "I just want to go home," I said. "I want to see my children." My words were choked with sobs, and I started to cry. But she walked over to the pictures of my daughters that I kept on the window and commented on how beautiful they were, and how much reason I had to get well. After some deep, calming breaths, I knew that to get through these dark times, I needed to constantly bring myself back to things that brightened my mood, like those beautiful children and the wholly unique and special wife who was waiting to spend the rest of my life with me. I realized that, as Baruch Spinoza said, "There is no hope unmingled with fear, and no fear unmingled with hope."

Find Your Points of Light

At these dark times, it is incumbent upon you to identify the points of light that help show *you* the way you need to go. There do not even need to be too many to make a significant difference in how you feel.

Do the following to demonstrate this. Stand in a completely pitch-black room. Now light a candle. Look around. Now the darkness is shattered, if not completely dissipated. How do you feel? There may be some scary spots around the edges of the limits or your candlelight, but the room does not really feel so frightening anymore, does it? You can see the outline of things, even recognize objects you know, and suddenly you feel more at ease in that room, maybe even comfortable.

Now use the candle you lit to light another candle. Note the difference it makes as the two candles supplement each other, each bringing their share of light and warmth to the once mysterious, unknown portions of the room that could not be seen before. Now use one of those candles to light a third. By now the once dark and forbidding room has a warm, almost joyous glow. Use those three candles to light three more. With six candles you may even have enough light to read or write. Each point of light you initiate not only makes a huge difference in chasing away the darkness but, like your candles, each can serve as the source of energy for the next one. Find one source of light and it will make it easier to find others.

If you are having trouble identifying your points of light, make a "list of blessings." Everyone has them. They can include your children and family, your friends, the fact that you have a job that allows you to pay the bills, the various, positive experiences you have had, and your best childhood memories. Then use this list to identify the things in life that you value most. Add to the list your "future blessings": the places you hope to visit, the family events you will attend, the anniversaries and birthdays you will celebrate. Those are your points of light. Organize them on your list and in your mind in a natural progression, for example, your child's next birthday, her sweet sixteen, her wedding day and the birth of your grandchildren. Each point of light will help illuminate the next one.

Seeing the Stars

Finding points of light can be done even in the most dire of circumstances. From the depths of Nazi persecution, Anne Frank wrote: "I don't think of all the misery but of the beauty that still remains." If a young girl who had everything taken away from her and was forced to live in fear could express these words, how much more so can we strive to think not of the misery of our cancer but rather of the beauty that still remains in our lives? Anne Frank simply had dreams and hopes that were greater to her than the difficulties she faced. You have to identify something that you love and long for more than you fear and hate your disease. Maybe it will be the faces of your children or your spouse. Perhaps it is a place you have visited or would like to visit. Focusing on those things will help you find your points of light.

Those points of light, however, are difficult to find if you are idle and not occupied in some way. There are several things you can try:

- When you are feeling down, move around. Do not wallow in loneliness in your room or house. If you are in the hospital, walk around and talk to people.
- Try to make others laugh (that will have a profound self-healing effect on you). As Mark Twain said, "The best way to cheer yourself up is to try to cheer somebody else up."
- If it is dangerous to be exposed to people, use your computer to chat with friends or family, or to tap into a support network of fellow patients.
- Do something fun. Watch a comedy routine (Chris Rock's "Bigger and Blacker" got me through some rough times). Listen to pleasant music. Play an instrument.

As Twain encouraged: "Drag your thoughts away from your troubles ... by the ears, by the heels, or any other way you can manage it." Even when you are feeling low, the very act of doing *something* to get you out of your funk will have the desired effect. Resist the temptation toward self-pity or the excuse that you simply feel too bad to do anything about it. Heed the words of Emory Austin: "Some days there won't be a song in your heart. Sing anyway."

If none of these activities helps you drag your thoughts away from your troubles and identify your points of light, reach out to someone you love or with whom you are comfortable speaking. There is a natural inclination among many people not to want to burden others. Some people feel like they need to always maintain a brave face. For these reasons, when times get rough, you may be hesitant to reach out to someone for support. Don't be. The people you love and who love you will not consider your need for companionship, attention, affection or a friendly ear to be a burden. To the contrary, they will probably appreciate being able to do something to help you along.

My lowest point during my treatment came about two and a half weeks into my first high-dose chemotherapy regimen. My white cell counts were almost nonexistent. I had no immunity. I would become feverish and shake like crazy. One Saturday, very early in the morning, my father, who, with my mother, was staying at the hospital over the Sabbath to keep me company, came to my room to see how I was doing. At that moment, I was all right and he left my room to say his morning prayers in the nearby visitors' lounge. Shortly afterward, I was given some medication to which I had a bad reaction. I started shaking terribly, to the point where I could not even breathe. The nurses put the side rails up on my bed and put me on oxygen. I whispered to them, "Get my father."

There I was, at thirty-three years old, a father of two myself, and I wanted my father with me because I was scared. He came in to be with me, rubbed my back and spoke quietly to me to try to calm me down. Finally, the nurse administered a shot of Demerol, the shaking subsided and I was able to breathe. I was exhausted and, as my father got up to finish his prayers and I was nodding off, I asked him to pray for me, because I simply did not have the strength to do it for myself.

Later on, when things had calmed down and the Sabbath was ending, my parents were getting ready to leave the hospital to head home and, although I was trying to put on my best brave face and assure them I was all right, silently I was hoping that my father would come back later and spend the night. He did not disappoint me. A couple of hours after he left, he returned with a bag and spent the night on the convertible chair-bed in my room. That night, after a couple of weeks of spiking fevers and frightening rigor, I woke up in a sweat. My fever had started to break. I like to think that the support and love I got from my father that night was my turning point from darkness into light. We never really outgrow the people we love, and they never really outgrow us. When you are at your lowest, trust them to raise you up.

Head It off at the Pass

To head off feelings of sadness, anxiety or fear in the first place, try to work calming activities into your schedule.

- If you are feeling worried or scared, discuss those feelings with someone you trust well before bedtime. Getting those feelings out can itself have a calming effect, essentially letting you unburden your mind of them for the time being.
- Avoid things that overstimulate the mind, especially with bad news. Do not watch television in the two hours or so preceding bedtime (and especially avoid the nightly news programs that are too often filled with violent and depressing imagery).
- Reduce the lighting in your room to enhance a relaxing mood.
- Listen to some soft, calming music. Music that incorporates nature sounds (a babbling brook, ocean waves or forest sounds) can be very soothing. What was written so long ago about music's calming effects remains true today: "Music has charms to calm the savage breast, to soften rocks or bend a knotted oak."[49] In fact, studies on the effect of music therapy on cancer patients suggest that listening to music can improve mood and an overall sense of well-being.[50] The positive effects of music on pain, stress and anxiety reduction have been demonstrated in studies on

---

49   William Congreve, *The Mourning Bride*, Act I, Scene I.

50   See, e.g., M. Barrera, "The effects of interactive music therapy on hospitalized children with cancer: a pilot study," *Psycho-Oncology*, vol. 11, no. 5 (September/October 2002), 378–388.

a variety of patient groups.[51] In my own treatment, I often used music to calm and distract me, particularly during bone marrow biopsies and chemotherapy treatments. I would listen to CDs that combined classical music with nature sounds, regulate my breathing and try to take my mind to "another place," someplace calm and serene. Although sometimes it was still difficult (there is only so much you can do when someone is sticking a needle into your hip bone), many times that approach made the process easier.

- Read an inspiring book or, if you are religiously inclined, identify specific biblical passages that lift your spirits, and recite them nightly before you go to bed. Meditate on the messages contained in these sources and how they apply to you.

Smells Good

If it does not affect any nausea symptoms you may be experiencing, use aromatherapy to induce restful sleep. Aromatherapy has been used for centuries for this and other purposes. Lavender oil has been associated in scientific studies with slowing activity of the nervous system and improving mood and sleep quality. For example, in a study conducted in Korea, female nursing students who complained of insomnia were exposed to lavender oil over a one-month period. Lavender aromatherapy was shown to reduce the amount of insomnia suffered by the study subjects

---

51   See R. Ulrich, "Effects of Healthcare Environmental Design on Medical Outcomes," *IADH*, International Academy for Design and Health (2001), 53; R. Hilliard, "Music Therapy in Hospice and Palliative Care: A Review of the Empirical Data," Evidence Based Complementary *Alternative Medicine* (June 2005): 2(2): 173–178 at pp. 175–176 (discussing studies that found that music therapy improved quality of life and mood, and reduced anxiety, among terminally ill patients).

and the amount of time it took them to fall asleep. Use of lavender oil also reduced depression in the study subjects.[52] In another study, exposure to lavender aroma was associated with reduced mental stress.[53]

Having a gentle massage with a solution of lavender oil may help you rest more completely. In fact, as discussed below, the healing effect of "touch" through massage has been demonstrated in several studies. Because some cancer treatments can make your skin sensitive, however, consult your doctor before using any oils or lotions on your skin. A good alternative is to sprinkle a couple of drops of lavender oil on your pillow at night or place a few drops of the oil into a container near your bed. Other essential oils that have been found to alleviate stress and promote relaxation include frankincense, sandalwood, jasmine, marjoram and rose.

Feels Good

That a "laying on of hands"—in other words, physical touch—can have beneficial healing effects has long been known and has been shown in several scientific studies. Deep-tissue pressure causes a release of endorphins (the "feel-good" hormone).[54] In fact, this positive effect of touch, and in particular massage, has been demonstrated repeatedly.

For example, a study undertaken at Memorial Sloan-Kettering Cancer Center followed 1,290 cancer patients receiving massage as part of their therapy over a three-year

---

52   I. S. Lee and G. J. Lee, "Effects of Lavender Aromatherapy on Insomnia and Depression in Women College Students," *Taehan Kanho Hakhoe Chi.* (February 2006); 36(1):136–143.

53   N. Motomura, et al., Reduction of Mental Stress with Lavender Odorant," *Percept Mot Skills* (December 2001): 93(3):713–718.

54   B. Kaada and O. Torsteinbo, "Increase of Plasma B-Endorphins in Connective Tissue Massage," *General Pharmacology: The Vascular System*, vol. 20, no. 4 (1989), 487–489.

period. The scores reported by patients in such areas as pain, fatigue, stress/anxiety, nausea and depression were 50 percent better among patients who received the massage therapy.[55] The Sloan-Kettering study noted that massage therapy was associated with greater pain management and reduction of nausea, anxiety and fatigue, as well as an enhanced sense of overall well-being.[56] Another study on 230 cancer patients found that massage therapy and healing touch were associated with reduced pain, fatigue and mood disturbance in patients receiving chemotherapy.[57] Aromatherapy coupled with massage also has been found to reduce anxiety and enhance overall well-being in cancer patients.[58]

You may have experienced the simple joy of touch or how hugs, a back rub or cuddling can improve your mood and give you an overall sense of well-being. As I mentioned earlier, my wife sometimes crawled into my hospital bed and cuddled with me to comfort me (and probably herself) and that was one of the best therapies I had during my entire treatment. The studies mentioned above explain why; those touches not only make you feel good emotionally but have positive biological effects. Those effects are especially important when you are experiencing the pain, anxiety or stress of cancer and its treatments. Utilize massage and healing touch to help you

---

55 B. Cassileth, PhD and A. Vickers, PhD, "Massage Therapy for Symptom Control: Outcome Study at a Major Cancer Center," *Journal of Pain and Symptom Management*, vol. 28, no. 3 (September 2004): 244–249 at 248.

56 Ibid., at 245.

57 J. Post-White, et al., "Therapeutic Massage and Healing Touch Improve Symptoms in Cancer," *Integrative Cancer Therapies* (2003): 2(4): 332–344 at 337–339, 343.

58 D. Fellowes, et al., "Aromatherapy and Massage for Symptom Relief in Patients with Cancer," *Cochrane Database of Systematic Reviews* (2008), issue 4. Art. No.: CD002287; doi:10.1002/14651858.CD002287.pub3.

alleviate the adverse effects of going through your cancer ordeal.

Your hospital may offer massage therapy as part of your cancer treatment. In the alternative, seek out a qualified massage therapist as a complement to your other cancer treatments. In addition, having healing touch or massage administered by someone you love can enhance the positive effects such therapy will have on you, as it will give you not only the biological benefits but also an increased feeling of being loved and supported.

Bear in mind, however, that your cancer treatments may make your skin, or at least certain areas on your body (for example, areas that have been exposed to radiation or have been operated on), very sensitive or sore. Make sure to advise anyone administering massage to you where these areas are. In addition, you should avoid massage over and around the area where a tumor is located. Also, make sure that you consult with your doctor to confirm that any oils or lotions you plan to use will not affect your skin or pose any other danger to you. Further, certain types of cancers (particularly leukemia) and cancer treatments can cause a drop in platelet counts and, as a result, massage can cause bruising. As such, as with all complementary treatments, consult your doctor to find out whether—and what type of—massage is good for you.

The people we love touch us in many ways; let their touch help you feel your way to health.

Looks Good: Seeing Yourself Well

Another good technique involves visualization. Record a message to yourself (or have someone you love do so) that includes the encouragement that you are going to be well. Repeat in that message that you are battling your cancer cells and destroying them. Remind yourself that you are doing everything in your power to rid your body of them. Include the message that all of your loved ones (reference them by name specifically) are supporting you and want you to be well. Tell yourself about the milestones you will celebrate in life after cancer (a child's wedding, a wedding anniversary, a long-delayed dream vacation). Play that recording on a low volume and concentrate on the messages you are giving yourself. In the same vein, create a mantra for yourself. It can be as simple as "I will be well," or "I will not let my cancer beat me," or "Every day I am a little bit stronger." Breathe deeply and repeat that mantra to yourself. Post it around your room for constant reminders.

As you employ these techniques, try as well to visualize your cancer in one way and the defenses of your body (your white blood cells and immune system) in another way. For example, you can envision your cancer cells in red and your healthy, cancer-fighting killer cells in white, and imagine the natural killer cells literally doing their job, blasting away the cancer cells. Another good image is to see your cancer cells as grains of black sand, and your healthy cells as the wind, rain or ocean waves, blowing or washing away those grains.

You can also imagine your cancer as a block of ice sitting outside, and your healthy cells or the medicine you are taking as the warm sun, melting away that block of ice and the resulting water running away from you. When you stand in the shower, visualize your cancer being washed away and swirling down the drain. (These visualizations also can be particularly helpful before you begin a treatment, as they will help you relax and may improve the efficacy of the treatment.) Utilizing such visualizations can both calm and empower you, as they will make you "see" your body ridding itself of your cancer. It functions almost as a form of self-hypnosis.

Indeed, there also is limited research associating positive visualization with a better clinical outlook for the patients who use it.[59] As the American Cancer Society has noted, several studies indicate that such visualization techniques can help manage stress, anxiety and depression, and may directly affect the immune system.[60]

One famous personality who insists that visualization allowed him to beat his bladder cancer is Academy Award–winning screenplay writer David Seidler, who wrote the screenplay for *The King's Speech*. Seidler underwent surgery to remove his initial bladder cancer in 2005, but forwent chemotherapy or removal of part of his bladder. He describes how, when his bladder cancer recurred some months later, he visualized his bladder as a "lovely, clean, healthy bladder." He said that he "spent hours visualizing a nice, cream-colored, unblemished bladder lining." His subsequent examination by his oncologist revealed that, incredibly, Seidler's cancer had disappeared. While such visualization may not help cure your cancer (and there is *significant debate* over whether it, in fact, can help do so), that it can have positive effects on your prognosis may be linked to the fact that it reduces stress and can put you in the frame of mind necessary to allow you to fight your cancer.

Remember the words of Napoleon Hill: "What the mind of man can believe and conceive, it can achieve."[61] If you conceive that you will be well, and believe that you will defeat your cancer, the dark hours will dissolve and you will be more likely to pursue and achieve your goal.

---

59 Gorter, *Fighting Cancer*, 260.

60 *Complete Guide*, 99.

61 N. Hill, *Think and Grow Rich*, 14.

CHAPTER 12

GIVE UP OR FIGHT LIKE HELL!

"If you're going through hell, keep going."
Winston Churchill

The road to your destination of health may have to pass through the fiery obstacles of chemotherapy, radiation or other difficult treatments. All of us who travel that road must make a conscious or subconscious decision to either allow ourselves to surrender or endeavor to remain dogged and determined. While perhaps his athletic achievements and championships have been called into doubt by his use of performance-enhancing drugs, Lance Armstrong's determination in defeating his cancer cannot be challenged. He wrote: "If children have the ability to ignore all odds and percentages, then maybe we can all learn from them. When you think about it, what other choice is there but to hope? We have two options, medically and emotionally: give up, or fight like hell."[62]

Many of my friends and relatives have commented on my high spirits in the face of my diagnosis and intensive treatment.

"How did you do it?" they ask.

---

62 L. Armstrong, *It's Not About the Bike: My Journey Back to Life*, 273.

"It was simple," I tell them. "When you have cancer, you have a choice. Either you can become despondent and expend your precious energy on self-pity, or you can resolve to," as Lance Armstrong said, "fight like hell." I made a conscious decision that I *would not* become despondent; that I would maintain my high spirits and make sure other people saw them; that I would hope for and believe in the best. I believed then, as I do now, that, as Winston Churchill said, "Attitude is a little thing that makes a big difference."

That hope and belief that you will be well can actually assist the healing process is borne out by the use of placebos in patients suffering from pain. Even patients who have been administered solutions containing no pain medication at all have experienced significant pain reduction when they were *told* that the injection they were receiving was a powerful pain reliever such as morphine. Again, although definitive, scientific proof that a positive attitude can dictate the course of a person's cancer is lacking, what the mind believes will happen may trigger a response in the body to try to *make* it happen, and what the mind believes will not happen may, in response, be prevented by the body from happening.

In *Everyone's Guide to Cancer Therapy*, the authors note that "[m]any physicians have seen how two patients of similar ages and with the same diagnosis, degree of illness, and treatment program experience vastly different results ... One of the few apparent differences is that one patient is pessimistic and the other optimistic."[63] They go on to relate the story of a patient who had recurrent breast cancer, which ultimately reached Stage IV and spread to her liver and bones. Her approach to her disease was as follows:

63 E. Rosenbaum, "The Will to Live," in M. Dollinger, et al., *Everyone's Guide to Cancer Therapy: How Cancer is Diagnosed, Treated, and Managed Day to Day*, 259 (4th ed. 2002).

I get out of bed every morning as if nothing was wrong … I may have known I was going to have to face things and could feel sick during the day, but I never got out of bed that way. There was a lot I was fighting for. I had a three-year-old child, a wonderful life, and a magical love affair with my husband.

Thirty years later, she was still alive and "still living an active life."[64]

That same frame of mind was brought home to me when a friend of mine, tongue-in-cheek, remarked to me as he was leaving my hospital room, "Don't die on me." I responded simply, "Not today." That became my personal mantra: "I am not going to die today." Every day I would repeat that mantra to myself, sometimes silently, sometimes out loud so I could not only think it but hear it. I repeatedly used my mind to convince myself and my body that I would not die. I *could not* die: I had too much to live for.

Although I did not conceptualize it at the time, that approach—what many people refer to simply as taking things "one day at a time"—is timeless. As the Bible relates Moses telling the Children of Israel: "See, I put before you *this day* life and good, death and evil."[65] He then exhorts the People to "choose life."[66] Moses was stressing something that is as true now as it was then: that *each day* we must choose life and determine how to live that life.

That is not to say that I never had low times, when I doubted my ability to recover or worried about whether I would ever see my children grow up. Such feelings are normal and, I would even say, inevitable. However, I was able consistently to bring myself back from those thoughts into positivity

---

64   Ibid., 260.

65   Deuteronomy 30:15.

66   Ibid., 30:19.

by seeing myself well and promising myself that I was "not going to die today", that I would "choose life" each day, and each day I did not die. While I may not have any conclusive scientific evidence to show that that positive mindset aided in my recovery, I feel sure that it did, and many other cancer survivors would relate similar beliefs.

Set Goals

A key to living up to that promise, and to fight my disease like hell, was to set both short-term and long-term goals for myself. Few things in life, including healing, or even living and dying, can be accomplished all at once. If I had to go through a bone marrow procedure, I would focus on the next five minutes, after which I knew it would be over. In terms of my treatment in the hospital, I marked off, both mentally and on a calendar, the number of days and chemotherapy injections I had left, each time making a mental strike through one of them. I kept in mind that each day marked off brought me one step closer to getting home.

This process is no different than conquering other obstacles. When you begin exercising, for example, focusing on the hour you are going to be on a treadmill, the miles you have left to run or the number of repetitions you have to do, may make your goal seem daunting or even unreachable. But when you focus instead on the next step, and the one after that and the one after that, each one becomes easier and brings you one step closer to your destination. Each repetition completed is one more behind you. Your cancer treatment is like a stairway. While your ultimate goal is to get to the top, do not look all the way up that stairway to your goal. Rather, view each step individually and focus on how each one has brought you closer to the top. Be realistic and pragmatic with yourself. Bear in mind that you may not be able to do as much all at once as you did before you started treatment.

At the same time, I also set longer-term goals for myself. Ending my immediate hospitalization was one. Getting through the first round of chemotherapy was another. Getting through chemotherapy maintenance, which was going to take most of a year, was a third. I also set personal goals beyond my cancer. The trip I promised my wife we would take when the cancer was gone was a driving force. We actually ultimately celebrated my remission and the end of my chemotherapy with a remarriage in Las Vegas and a second honeymoon in Hawaii, things we always hoped to be able to do. Our friends arranged a remarriage celebration when we returned. Even longer-term goals than those, including seeing my daughters and dancing with them at their bat mitzvahs and weddings, also became part of my plan. Setting and marking off the realization of such goals will give you something to constantly look forward to and give you a more tangible sense of progress as you move through your treatments.

Find Your "Why" (Part Two)

Visualizing these goals and actually scheduling them played a significant role in getting me through some difficult times. In chapter 2, I discussed the importance of finding your *why* in the context of "Why has this happened to me?" at the outset of your cancer journey. Finding your "why" early on in your cancer battle can help ease your mind and focus your plan of attack and defense.

Now that you are in the throes of treatment and recovery, your "why" becomes relevant in a related context. Nietzsche wrote that: "He who has a why to live can bear almost any how." In other words, if you can identify and stay focused on what it is you want to accomplish—your *why* when it comes to fighting through your treatment to your ultimate goal —you will be better able to endure *how* you get there.

So ask yourself: "Why should I keep pushing through this? What do I have to live for that makes the ordeal of cancer treatment worth it?"

Perhaps one of the best examples of this approach is a story related by Rabbi Berel Wein in his book *Buy Green Bananas*. Rabbi Wein writes about a friend who explained to him how he survived the Nazi death camp at Auschwitz, when others, many of whom were stronger than he, did not:

> In 1932, as a young, well-to-do businessman from Budapest, I went on a trip to the Holy Land. I was so enamored of the country that I bought a house in Jerusalem on the spur of the moment. I usually never allowed my emotions to rule my behavior, let alone my wallet, but this time I acted impulsively and out of character. The house was badly in need of refurbishing, so I hired an architect to draw up the necessary plans to redesign and rebuild the dwelling. I then became absorbed in other business projects, and I never actually had time to follow up on the plans or the renovation. However, every night in Auschwitz, while lying together with 13 other human beings on a plank of wood that was the width of a king-size bed, after a day of labor and humiliation, pain and death, with my senses numbed by hunger, lice and filth, I imagined how I was going to rebuild that Jerusalem apartment of mine. I furnished and refurnished it every night in my imagination. I moved walls and opened windows, and every night I imagined it differently. That is how I survived those 10 months in Auschwitz. That is how I saved my sanity and my Jewish faith.[67]

Focus on what you want to achieve both during and after your cancer treatments. Use your list of blessings and points

---

67 Rabbi Berel Wein, *Buy Green Bananas*, 176–177.

of light to guide you. See those things clearly and plan them carefully and in detail. See yourself celebrating those goals. Establish your *why* to survive and *how* you do so will be secondary.

CHAPTER 13

APPRECIATE GOOD PEOPLE

"Genuinely good people are like that. The sun shines out of them. They warm you right through."
Michael Morpurgo, *Alone on a Wide Wide Sea*

It is too easy when we are dealing with cancer to feel embittered and irritated. After all, the specter of what might happen to us if our treatments do not work, as well as the grueling effects of going through them, can simply make things hard to deal with. You may become annoyed and short-tempered. It is very easy in these circumstances to fail to recognize the good that is done for you not only by your friends and relatives but by essential strangers. There will probably be many such people who play a critical role in your convalescence.

Whereas a good doctor is worth her weight in gold, a good nurse is priceless. For as much as you may rely on your doctor to guide you through your treatment and keep you up to date on your progress, if you spend any time at all in the hospital it will be the nurses who actually interact with and care for you. Nurses often see you at your worst when you are being treated for cancer. They may see you naked, watch you lose your hair, change your soiled bedding or clean your bedpans, help you shower, make sure you are eating properly and dispense your medication. In short, they will be the medical personnel on whom you rely most heavily. They will be the ones who are there in the night when visiting hours have ended and you are feeling down. They have to function both as medical professionals and psychologists. Too often their contributions to patient care get second recognition to that of the oncologists who diagnose and prescribe the treatment for cancer. Yet they are healers in every sense of the word.

In my own case, the nurses who handled me during my hospitalization were beyond words in their commitment to the patients in my ward. Granted, inasmuch as I was in a dedicated leukemia ward, the nurses were acclimated to patients who had to spend a lot of time in the hospital and, as such, I would imagine that that position weeded out people who were not very good at communicating with and comforting their patients. I, in turn, always endeavored to treat them with humor and respect. I shared the goodies friends and family brought to me with the nursing staff. I made a point of thanking them each time they did something for me, even if it was just taking my blood pressure or drawing my blood. I saw too many justifiably frustrated and frightened patients or their families lash out at nurses or unjustifiably treat them with some degree of contempt, however. I recall one patient in particular who became frustrated with his nurse's instructions as to how he needed to administer certain injections to himself at home as part of his treatment. As his frustration mounted he finally blurted out, "Look, who's dying here, me or you?"

Remember that your nurses are not actually *your* nurses. They have any number of other patients to whom to attend, probably at the very moment that you want them to do something for you. If they do not respond immediately to a call, it will not be because they are lazy at responding or simply inattentive to your needs. They *care*. If they did not, they would not be doing what they do. If they cannot do more for you than you want, remember that they are limited in some respects by what your doctor directs. Treat them well, as ultimately they will wind up giving a great amount to you—kindness, encouragement and support—over the course of your treatment.

There is also an array of other support personnel in the hospital who may fly under your radar. Volunteers, candy stripers, orderlies, physicians assistants, custodians, etc., all play a vital role in your hospital care, whether it be by bringing your meals, cleaning your room and bathroom (often under less than pleasant circumstances), changing your bedding, bringing you reading material or simply offering support. Even people on the administrative end who get you admitted and help you with your paperwork are doing a service to help simplify your complex situation. Some of these people are not even being paid for their time, but volunteer out of their desire to do good things for their fellow man. Do not dismiss them. Appreciate them and how much they do to make your ordeal more comfortable. Get their names and send a letter to the hospital extolling the contributions and virtues of these underappreciated angels.

PART III

LEAVE NO STONE UNTURNED
Complementing Your Cancer Treatments

CHAPTER 14

EATING WELL TO BE WELL

"Let thy food be thy medicine and thy medicine thy food."
Hippocrates

Hippocrates' admonition to let medicine be our food and let food be our medicine expresses the belief that getting proper nutrition can help your body heal. If you are going through chemotherapy or radiation, however, or are about to or have just finished a round of it, or if you are recovering from surgery, eating may be the furthest thing from your mind (and the least pleasant thought when you *can* think about it). That feeling can result from several factors: the inability to keep food down that chemotherapy and radiation often bring on; anxiety over your condition or treatment; or simple lack of appetite brought on by your disease, treatment or fatigue.

In my case, although my stomach handled the chemotherapy relatively well, with few bouts of true nausea and some diarrhea, my difficulty in eating grew out of my simple inability to taste anything. Chemotherapy had, quite simply, killed my sense of taste, as it does for many patients, and, as a result, eating held no charm for me. All I could really taste were the extremes; either very salty or very sweet. As such, most of my diet during my month-long initial hospitalization consisted of saltines and tuna or my mother's chicken soup, which she prepared and brought to me regularly. Chicken soup? Yes, I know it is a cliché, but some clichés do come from some factual basis and, in my case, that protein-laden soup truly sustained me. Other than those items, however, eating was really a chore. I simply resolved to eat because I knew it was important to keep up my strength.

Still, I had very little guidance at the time as to what I should be eating—or not eating—to help me defeat my cancer and make the most of my treatments. Let me preface what will follow in this chapter with the same type of caveat I have given earlier in other contexts. The precise role that proper nutrition plays in getting cancer—or getting rid of it—is not settled definitively. While for some cancers (particularly digestive tract and colorectal cancers), there is reasonably strong epidemiological and other evidence to suggest a link between consumption of certain types of foods and cancer incidence, for most cancers the role of nutrition—and the roles of specific foods or food derivatives—in either causing or helping to cure cancer is still being debated (and even for cancers for which there *are* stronger dietary-based links, there are also other potential causes and confounding factors).

Moreover, while I cite several studies to support the associations between certain dietary habits (such as consumption of excess sugar, meat and processed foods) and the promotion of cancer, or others that discuss how certain dietary approaches (i.e., focusing on whole, unprocessed and plant-based foods) may impede the growth of cancer cells or help destroy them, there are also many studies that either refute or fail to replicate the findings in the ones I cite. Much of what has been promoted regarding the anti-cancer effects of certain foods comes from animal or laboratory studies—that are controlled strictly for confounding factors and are difficult to apply to human experience in the absence of confirmatory epidemiological data—or anecdotal human experience.

Thus, while I believe that, ultimately, what we eat or drink can affect whether we get—or get rid of—cancer, it is not the goal of this chapter to *prove* that. Rather, the information I am presenting here is designed to raise that possibility. If, in fact, these nutritional approaches can help you defeat your cancer, what you will gain by following them will be substantial (at minimal cost to you). Even if they do not directly affect the progression or defeat of your cancer, however, these approaches can provide other advantages in your cancer fight— namely, increased energy, a potential lessening of treatment side effects and a greater sense of control over your plan of attack. I encourage you, therefore, to approach the information and suggestions in this chapter with an open mind, a discerning eye and, if you will excuse the pun, a grain of salt.

That having been said, eating as properly as possible, and getting sufficient nutrition, when you are going through cancer treatments is vital. A soldier on the battlefield faces physical obstacles and pushes his body past all natural barriers to fatigue. As a result, getting enough nutrition is crucial for an effective fighting force (hence the maxim that an army marches on its stomach). We, fighting the battle against cancer, and putting our bodies through the hell of conventional cancer treatments, are not unlike those soldiers. We are waging our war against a vicious enemy, and we need the energy to fight that battle. Insufficient nutrition may lead to a weakened immune system and decreased disease resistance.

Yet there are proper and improper ways to approach nutrition during—and even after—your cancer ordeal. Cancer incidence has increased substantially in Western countries over the past seventy years or so. While there are several potential explanations for this increase (such as increased exposure to environmental toxins and increased overall life expectancy, which allows for cancers with long latency periods to develop), and it is impossible to pin the blame for this increased incidence on any one factor, significant changes in dietary routines and the food we eat in that period are among the suspected causes.

For example, there has been a tremendous increase in the amount of sugar consumed in the typical Western diet, and foods, including both plant and animal sources, have undergone a significant amount of engineering, through pesticide use and genetic modification. The amount of man-made additives going into our food sources has increased dramatically as well. Asian countries, which for years had a lower incidence of many cancers than Western nations, have seen their cancer rates increase as Western dietary trends (including fatty fast food and sugar-laden foods) have infiltrated their societies. As such, avoiding those types of foods—which, in any event, provide lower quality nutrition than the other types of foods discussed below—and revamping your diet may play a role in improving your health and helping you defeat your cancer.

If, like me, you have well-meaning, loving friends and families, you undoubtedly will receive gifts of candy, cookies, brownies, etc. Don't indulge in them. Give them to the nursing staff or the orderlies who are such a huge help in our times of weakness. You may have heard the oft-repeated—although overly simplistic—mantra that "sugar feeds cancer." This belief stems from the fact that, while all cells use glucose to produce energy for the body, cancer cells consume much more glucose than normal cells.[68] Indeed, PET scans, which are often used to detect cancer, in fact identify areas in the body in which glucose is being consumed in the largest amounts (i.e., often where cancer cells are active).[69]

---

68 See "Does Sugar Feed Cancer," http://www.sciencedaily.com/releases/2009/08/090817184539.htm (describing a study undertaken at the Huntsman Cancer Institute at the University of Utah evaluating the role of sugar and glutamine in cancer cell growth).

69 See *Anticancer*, 61.

The association between sugar consumption and cancer, however, is more complex. In addition to leading to obesity, which is itself a risk factor for certain types of cancers, excess sugar intake can trigger the production of higher amounts of insulin and insulin-like growth factor-1 ("IGF-1"). Insulin and IGF-1, in effect, "rev up" cell growth. They also may enhance the ability of cancer cells to invade surrounding tissue.[70] While ramping up cell growth is good in the context of healthy cells, when you are fighting cancer you want to avoid revving up your cancer cells and feeding their growth through the production of excess insulin.

Therefore, to limit this potential effect, restrict your sugar intake to natural sugars found in fruits and natural-sourced carbohydrates (sweet potatoes, brown rice and vegetables), and keep your intake of sugary fruits and carbohydrates to a minimum. When you do consume these natural sugars, combine them with other foods that provide healthy fats (such as nuts, avocados, seeds and olive oil), proteins (beans, peas, lentils and quinoa) and fiber (whole grains and brown rice), which help regulate the amount of insulin your body produces. Avoid foods made with white flour, such as most breads and pasta, as consumption of white flour also can cause a spike in blood sugar levels. The goal of this approach is to avoid creating conditions in your body that might make cancer cells multiply or more resistant to your treatment.[71] At a minimum, following a dietary approach that helps you maintain a more even blood sugar level will give you the sustained energy necessary to help you deal with your treatments and engage as much as possible in the rest of your life activities.

---

70 Ibid.

71 For a general discussion of this issue and a list of studies addressing the alleged sugar-cancer link, see, e.g., "Sugar and Cancer: Is There a Connection," http://www.caring4cancer.com/go/cancer/nutrition/questions/sugar-and-cancer-is-there-a-connection.htm.

Instead of pre-packaged or processed foods, seek your nourishment from simple, natural, unprocessed foods. As Jack LaLanne, the grandfather of modern physical fitness, used to say, "If man made it, don't eat it." In other words, if it grew or moved on its own (and was not genetically modified), it is a candidate for being eaten. If it was made in a laboratory, avoid it. That philosophy, coupled with a lifetime of regular exercise, served Jack LaLanne well. He passed away at ninety-six, and was the picture of good health for all of his adult life.

As a general rule of thumb, the fewer ingredients a food product has, the more likely it is that it does not contain potentially damaging man-made food additives. If the list of ingredients is several inches long and includes a lot of things you cannot identify (and contains words with many syllables), avoid it. Even among "healthy" choices of fruits and vegetables, seek out organic produce that has not been treated with pesticides or genetically modified. Also, as much as possible, control the origin of your food. In other words, make it fresh and make it yourself. If other people are preparing food for you, do not be bashful about giving them directions as to what you can and cannot eat. Getting proper nutrition during your treatment not only supports healthy tissues but may help your body battle and destroy cancer cells.

Since eating may be a chore for you, stick to simple foods that are easy for the body to break down but are high in nutritional value. Focus on:

- Fish that contain oils high in omega-3 fatty acids eicosapentaenoic acid (EPA) and docosahexaenoic acid (DHA), which some research suggests may decrease cancer cells' ability to attach themselves to blood vessels. Several fish species, including mackerel, salmon, herring, sardines, sablefish (black cod), anchovies and albacore tuna contain these healthy fats. Due to environmental pollution, however, some of these fish species may also contain high levels of heavy metals or other contaminants, so be conscious of this issue when choosing what type of fish to include in your diet and the sources of those fish. One alternative is to seek these nutrients from plant sources, such as flaxseeds, which are another potent source of omega-3 fatty acids and can easily be incorporated into meals by being sprinkled on salads or cereals. Animal and laboratory studies—which, again, may not be directly applicable to humans—suggest that consuming such foods may help reduce inflammation and the risk of metastasis (the spread of cancer) from one site in the body to others, and slow tumor growth.[72] If you are not eating, or cannot eat, fish, ask your doctor which supplements are available to give you these nutrients and whether those supplements are right for you.

---

72 See, e.g., D. P. Rose, et al., "Diet and Breast Cancer," American Institute for Cancer Research, Plenum Press, 1994, 83–91; Y. Shao, et al., "Enhancement of the Antineoplastic Effect of Mitomycin C by Dietary Fat," *Cancer Res.* (1994): 54: 6452–6457; Y. Shao, et al., "Dietary Menhaden Oil Enhances Mitomycin C Antitumor Activity Toward Human Mammary Carcinoma MX-1," *Lipids* 30 (1995): 1035–1045. One cautionary note, however, is that certain studies have actually found an *increased* risk of prostate cancer associated with omega-3 levels. See T. Brasky, et al., "Serum Phospholipid Fatty Acids and Prostate Cancer Risk: Results from the Prostate Cancer Prevention Trial," *American Journal of Epidemiology* (2011): 173 (12) 1429–1439; T. Brasky, et al., "Plasma Phospholipid Fatty Acids and Prostate Cancer Risk" in the SELECT Trial, JNCI J. Natl Cancer Inst (2013): 10.1093/jnci/djt174. In contrast, other studies have found that certain types of fatty acids may increase the risk of prostate cancer but that omega-3 was associated with lower prostate cancer risks. See M. Leitzmann, et al., "Dietary Intake of n-3 and n-6 Fatty Acids and the Risk of Prostate Cancer," *American Journal of Clinical Nutrition* 80 (2004) 204–216. As with all dietary changes, therefore, consult with your doctor before undertaking them.

- Foods high in fiber, such as unrefined whole grains (including, for example, brown rice and oat bran), beans, peas, nuts, spinach, acorn squash, figs and dates. Several of these food sources also contain substantial amounts of protein. Fiber-rich foods help the body maintain more constant blood sugar levels. They also promote a healthy excretory process, which will help rid your body of many toxins and may alleviate some of the gastrointestinal difficulties associated with conventional cancer treatments. In fact, if you have been raised on a diet that included white rice over brown rice varieties and was deficient in raw, natural fruits and vegetables, you will be amazed at just how good these foods taste and how fulfilling they can be. High-protein foods also help maintain an even blood sugar level. Organic meats, poultry and fish are possible choices, but bear in mind that animal proteins take longer to digest than plant proteins. As a result, it will take longer for the nutrients in such foods to reach your cells and longer for the leftover waste and toxins from them to be excreted. In addition, if chemotherapy has made it difficult for you to keep food down, animal proteins may not be the best choice. Plant-based proteins, such as lentils, peas, beans and quinoa are good choices and often can be included in soups, which are easier to eat and digest. These foods also contain phytochemicals, which some people believe are effective in fighting cancer. Thus, for example, the American Cancer Society notes that: "There is some evidence that certain phytochemicals may help prevent the formation of potential carcinogens (substances that cause cancer), block the action of carcinogens on their target organs or tissue, or act on cells to suppress cancer development. Many experts suggest that people can reduce their risk of cancer significantly by eating more fruits, vegetables, and other foods from plants that contain phytochemicals."[73] In fact, countries in which the average diet is high in these types of foods have been shown to have lower rates of certain cancers than countries in which there is a higher consumption of meat and dairy products.[74] Further, some research suggests that a diet that eliminates or significantly restricts the intake of animal-based proteins may retard the growth of certain types of cancer cells.[75] In one such study, ninety-three patients who had been diagnosed with prostate cancer who had chosen not to undergo surgery to remove their cancer, or other clinical treatment, were followed for one year. One group of the study subjects was monitored without changing their lifestyles. The other group was prescribed a regimen that included a vegetarian diet, exercise (walking thirty minutes a day), vitamin supplements and stress management techniques. The study demonstrated that whereas the cancer of several patients in the "do nothing" group worsened, resulting in them needing surgery and/ or chemotherapy or radiation, none of the patients in the second group needed such treatment.[76] PSA levels in the

---

73   American Cancer Society, "Phytochemicals" at http://www.cancer. org/Treatment/TreatmentsandSideEffects/ComplementaryandAlternativeMedicine/HerbsVitaminsandMinerals/phytochemicals.

74   *Anticancer*, 73. See also D. Ornish, et al., "Intensive Lifestyle Changes May Affect the Progression of Prostate Cancer," *174 Journal of Urology*, no. 3 (September 2005), 1065–1070 at 1065 ("Ornish") (prostate cancer lower in countries where the predominant diet is plant-based and low-fat); D. Alberts and L. Loescher, "Cancer Prevention, Screening, and Risk Assessment," in *Everyone's Guide to Cancer*," 329 ("Populations that consume large amounts of plant-derived foods have decreased incidence of certain types of cancers," including esophageal, mouth, stomach, colon, rectum, lung and prostate cancers).

75   See, for example, Campbell and Campbell, *The China Study*, 348–349, 367.

76   Ornish, *supra*, 1067.

"do nothing" group increased, whereas levels in the experimental group decreased.[77] Moreover, the blood of the patients in the revised lifestyle group was demonstrated to be *eight times more capable* of restricting the growth of cancer cells.[78] Thus, a diet high in fruits, vegetables and dietary fiber may "have the ability to short-circuit development of [certain] cancers."[79] The sufficiency of a properly balanced vegetarian diet also was confirmed in the United States Department of Agriculture's 2010 Dietary Guidelines for Americans, which noted that meat consumption is not essential and that vegetarian (or near-vegetarian) diets may, in fact, be protective against certain types of cancer and healthier overall than diets that include meat.[80]

- Mushrooms: Certain ingredients found in mushrooms may stimulate the immune system. Several studies on the potential immune-enhancing effects of mushroom consumption have been undertaken in Japan, where mushrooms play a large role in the national diet. Those studies have found, among other things, that patients who are given mushroom extracts show an increase in the amount and activity of immune cells and that certain types of mushrooms largely prevent the growth of cancer cells in in vitro (laboratory) studies.[81] Other animal and laboratory studies have identified certain types of mushrooms as being effective against esophageal, stomach, prostate and lung cancers.[82] The anti-tumorigenic effects seen in

---

77 Ibid., 1068.

78 Ibid., 1065.

79 *Everyone's Guide to Cancer*, 330.

80 USDA Dietary Guidelines for Americans, 35, 45.

81 *Anticancer*, 106.

82 A. S. Daba and O. U. Ezeronye, "Anti-Cancer Effects of Polysaccharides Isolated From Higher Basidiomycetes Mushrooms," *African Journal of Biotechnology*, vol. 2(12) (December 2003): 672–678 at 673.

such studies may be linked to the role of mushrooms in boosting immune function.[83] Lentinan, a component found in shiitake mushrooms, has been associated with slowed tumor growth, as well as prolonged cancer survival, particularly in patients with gastric and colorectal cancers.[84] In addition, the meaty texture of many mushrooms makes them a welcome addition to the plates of patients who have eliminated meat from their diet. While their nutritional benefits are greatest when raw, mushrooms can be prepared in various ways that create opportunities for interesting changes to your daily menu. They can be grilled, sautéed, used in soups or salads or even dehydrated and eaten as a snack.

- Avoiding foods that increase inflammation in the body, such as fatty foods (particularly foods with trans fats), vegetable oils (such as sunflower, corn and soy oil), food that includes white flour and processed sugar, fried foods, dairy, red meat and alcohol.

- Consuming foods that contain high levels of antioxidants, such as fruits, berries, vegetables and walnuts, especially after your chemotherapy treatments have started. Antioxidants may protect against the type of genetic damage that some researchers believe plays a role in cancer progression.[85] Green tea is a great source of antioxidants (called catechins), is believed by some people to help prevent metastasis and has been associated with lower cancer incidence and recurrence rates. The antioxidants in green tea scavenge on free radicals, which can damage

---

83   Ibid., 673–674, 676.

84   Ibid., 674–675.

85   *Everyone's Guide to Cancer*, 330.

DNA and perhaps thereby promote cancerous growth.[86] Polyphenols found in green tea have been observed in laboratory studies to slow the growth of leukemia, and breast, prostate, kidney, skin and mouth cancer.[87] The National Cancer Institute has noted that, although human studies have been inconclusive, "tea and/or tea poly- phenols have been found in animal studies to inhibit tu- morigenesis at different organ sites including the skin, oral cavity, esophagus, stomach, small intestine, colon, liver, pancreas and mammary gland."[88] Laboratory studies have indicated that green tea "inhibits breast cancer growth by a direct anti-proliferative effect on the tumor cells.[89] The *Carcinogenesis* study also indicated that green tea consumption increased the effectiveness of tamoxifen, a drug used commonly to treat breast cancer.[90] Further, green tea helps the body eliminate toxins and, like other antioxidant foods, helps reduce bodily inflammation that some researchers contend promotes the growth of cancer cells.[91] Still, the variance of findings in studies on the health benefits of green tea has led the Food and Drug

---

86　See S. M. Hennings, "Bioavailability and Antioxidant Activity of Tea Flavanols After Consumption of Green Tea, Black Tea and Green Tea Extract Supplement," *American Journal of Clinical Nutrition* (2004): 80(6):1558–1564.

87　*Anticancer*, 102.

88　"Tea and Cancer Prevention: Strengths and Limits of the Evidence," at http://www.cancer.gov/cancertopics/factsheet/prevention/tea.

89　M. Sartippour, et al. "The Combination of Green Tea and Tamoxifen is Effective Against Breast Cancer," *Carcinogenesis* (2006): 27(12):2424–2433, 2424.

90　Ibid., 2431.

91　Ibid.; E. H. Byun, et al., "TLR4 Signaling Inhibitory Pathway Induced by Green Tea Polyphenol Epigallocatechin-3-Gallate through 67-kDa Laminin Receptor," *Journal of Immunology* 185, no. 1 (July 2010) 33–45 (discussing the anti-inflammatory effects of constituents of green tea).

Administration to conclude that such beneficial effects have not been proven conclusively.[92]

- Consuming several servings of green, leafy vegetables. Spinach, kale, romaine lettuce, collards and parsley are particularly good sources of minerals (such as iron, potassium, calcium and magnesium) and vitamins (including vitamins B, C, E and K). They also include cell-protecting nutrients such as lutein and beta-carotene. They are low in fat and high in dietary fiber. Kale is among the highest antioxidant vegetables and also has inflammation-regulating properties. If you find that it is difficult to eat and/or digest these vegetables while you are undergoing treatment, get yourself a good vegetable juicer or blender and make green juice or smoothies instead. (If you have never "juiced" before, juices or smoothies containing only green vegetables can taste pretty intense. Add sweeter vegetables, such as carrots or beets, or an apple or berries, to sweeten the juice if necessary, but remember to limit your sugar intake).

- Cruciferous vegetables: Cruciferous vegetables, such as broccoli, Brussels sprouts, cauliflower and cabbage contain compounds called isothiocyanates. One such isothiocyanate, sulforathane (SFN), is found in high levels in broccoli and, in even higher amounts, in broccoli sprouts (which can often be found in the salad or vegetable section of your supermarket and contain eight to ten times the SFN found in broccoli florets).[93] Several studies undertaken in the laboratory setting suggest that SFN may be an effective chemopreventive agent, which

---

92 See the FDA's June 30, 2005, press release at http://www.fda.gov/news-events/newsroom/pressannouncements/2005/ucm108452.htm.

93 See J. Finley, et al., "Cancer-Protective Properties of High Selenium Broccoli," *Journal of Agricultural Food Chemistry* (2001): 49, 2679–2683 at 2679, 2682.

aids in blocking the initiation of cancer cell production and suppressing their growth, thereby helping to delay the development of or shorten the survival time of cancer cells, as well as helping the body eliminate carcinogenic toxins.[94] SFN has been shown in such studies to target pancreatic cancer cells.[95] Several epidemiological studies indicate that people who consume cruciferous vegetables have lower risks of prostate, lung, breast and colon cancers.[96] So, do what your mother always told you: Eat your broccoli (and other vegetables).

- Wheatgrass juice: Ann Wigmore was the pioneer of the use of wheatgrass juice for therapeutic purposes, and the creator of the Hippocrates Health Institute (HHI), which promotes the use of wheatgrass juice and a raw vegan diet, as well as exercise and stress relief, in the treatment of disease and to further a healthy lifestyle. Proponents of wheatgrass juice extol the many potential health benefits of drinking a few ounces of it each day (although critics dispute the extent to which wheatgrass consumption promotes better health). Wheatgrass has an extremely high amount of chlorophyll, which may give it a very energizing and alkalizing effect. It is an excellent source of vitamins C, E, K and B complex (including B12), and is rich in minerals such as calcium, cobalt, germanium, iron, magnesium, phosphorus, potassium, protein, sodium, sulphur and zinc. Further, wheatgrass contains some seventeen

---

94 See M. Myzak and R. Dashwood, "Chemoprevention by Sulforathane: Keep One Eye Beyond Keap1," Cancer Lett. (February 28, 2006): 233(2):208–218, at 208–209 ("Myzak"); Y. Li, et al., "Sulforathane, a Dietary Component of Broccoli/Broccoli Sprouts, Inhibits Breast Cancer Stem Cells," Clin Cancer Res, 16(9) (May 1, 2010): 2580–2590 at 2580, 2586 ("Li").

95 Ibid., 2581.

96 Myzak, supra, and studies cited therein; Li, 2583–2586.

types of amino acids and approximately eighty enzymes. The high alkalinity and antioxidant characteristics of wheatgrass also give it anti-inflammatory properties and help fight free radicals in the body, which, as discussed, may be associated with the body's ability to fight cancer. As the authors of one study that investigated the effects of wheatgrass juice consumption on patients with APL— the same cancer I had—noted, wheatgrass juice "contains most of the vitamins and minerals needed for human maintenance."[97] This study indicated, again, only in the laboratory setting, that wheatgrass consumption may be toxic to certain types of leukemia cells.[98] The study authors noted that the active component in wheatgrass appears to restrict the metabolic activity of cancer cells.[99] Moreover, although wheatgrass was associated with cytotoxic and nonproliferative effects on *leukemia* cells, it did not show these effects on *healthy* cells.[100] Further, a study undertaken at the University of California, Berkeley, found that consumption of wheatgrass juice by breast cancer patients during their course of chemotherapy helped alleviate some of the side effects of their treatment. These patients demonstrated a decreased need for blood and bone marrow building medications during their treatment, without lessening the effects of their chemotherapy.[101] Patients in the study who drank wheatgrass juice during the course of

---

97 N. B. Alitheen, *et al.*, "Cytotoxic Effects of Commercial Wheatgrass and Fiber Towards Human Acute Promyelocytic Leukemia Cells (HL60)," *Pak J Pharm Sci.* (July 2011): 24(3):243–50 at 243.

98 Ibid.

99 Ibid., 243.

100 Ibid., 249–250.

101 G. Bar-Sela, et al., "Wheat Grass Juice May Improve Hematological Toxicity Related to Chemotherapy in Breast Cancer Patients: A Pilot Study," *Nutrition and Cancer*, vol. 58, no. 1 (2007), 43–48 at 47.

chemotherapy experienced lower levels of hematological toxicity associated with their treatment.[102] They also experienced a lower incidence of neutropenic infections (infections linked to low white blood cell counts) and fever.[103] The study authors attributed these effects to the presence of apigenin, an anti-inflammatory flavonoid found in wheatgrass.[104] The researchers also theorized that chlorophyllin in wheatgrass, which has been shown to protect mitochondria in other circumstances, may also protect against the cellular damage caused by chemotherapeutic drugs.[105] The taste and smell of wheatgrass juice can be strong (think of how it smells right after you mow the lawn), but good, fresh wheatgrass juice has a sweetish taste and, just like the vegetables you hated to eat when you were younger because of the taste, the benefits of consuming wheatgrass juice may outweigh any momentary unpleasantness.

- Hydration: As a rule of thumb, drink half your weight in ounces each day. In other words, if you weigh 150 pounds, drink 75 ounces of healthy liquids daily. These liquids may include filtered water, green vegetable juices, green tea and homemade soups. (Just make sure substantial sugars or other harmful ingredients such as MSG have not been added to the soup. Someone who loves you can prepare homemade vegetable, lentil or pea soups that will be tasty, easy to get down and nutritious.)

- Eating smaller meals: When eating and keeping down what you eat are difficult, eating smaller amounts of food is the best approach. Try to eat several small meals during the course of the day rather than a few larger ones. This

---

102 Ibid., 45–46.

103 Ibid., 46.

104 Ibid.

105 Ibid.

will help reduce the nausea that may come from trying to digest a large amount of food, help maintain a more constant blood sugar level and provide more sustained energy (eating several smaller meals throughout the day actually boosts your metabolism). It may also help you identify specific foods that are more difficult for you to tolerate than others.[106]

The potential cancer-fighting benefits of various properly used food sources have been investigated extensively in human, animal and laboratory studies. The evidence as to whether or how certain food or food derivatives may help prevent or fight different types of cancers, while far from definitive, suggests that incorporating them into your diet may be a helpful complement to your other cancer treatments. As a 2003 article in *Nature* and other studies have noted: "Chemoprevention by edible phytochemicals is now considered to be an inexpensive, readily applicable, acceptable and accessible approach to cancer control and management."[107]

---

106 For a more in-depth discussion of the nutritional approach to fighting cancer, see generally: Gorter, *Fighting Cancer*, 148–153 (and studies cited therein; this book focuses on Dr. Gorter's immune-based approach to cancer treatment and includes a detailed discussion for understanding how cancer affects the body and the various approaches to treating it); *Anticancer*, 119–130; M. Keane and D. Chace, *What to Eat if You Have Cancer: Healing Foods that Boost Your Immune System* (this is a comprehensive book written by a cancer survivor that describes, in detail, how cancer attacks the body on the cellular level and how proper nutrition can help repair it, as well providing practical ideas for structuring your meals while you are undergoing chemotherapy or radiation treatments); R. Beliveau and D. Gingras, *Foods that Fight Cancer*.

107 Young-Joon Surh, "Cancer Chemoprevention with Dietary Phytochemicals," *Nature*, vol. 3 (October 2003): 768–780 at 777.

Some patients—including several I met at HHI—choose to treat their cancer using proper nutrition (in addition to exercise, stress management and other techniques discussed in this book), and forego conventional cancer treatments, such as chemotherapy and radiation. *This approach is not without risks and remains controversial.* Whether such an approach is right for you is something you should determine in consultation with your oncologist and a qualified nutritionist. No one diet or series of dietary suggestions—including the ones here—is right for everyone.

While dietary improvement may not be a magic bullet, and simply consuming more vegetables or avoiding harmful, inflammatory foods may not alone cure your cancer, these approaches can add critical weapons in your cancer-fighting arsenal, inasmuch as, at a minimum, they can help increase your strength and endurance, give you more control over how you feel and, thereby, decrease your stress and improve your mood. As noted in *Everyone's Guide to Cancer*:

> Good nutrition can increase immunity, promote feelings of well-being and a better mood, achieve better results of treatment and increase the quality of your life. Good nutrition enables you to have more energy to do the things you enjoy and love.[108]

Moreover, if you are someone who has grown up consuming a lot of processed foods and have not really investigated the world of natural food sources, recreating your diet can add exciting variety and discovery to your days. Use your cancer as an opportunity to open up your palate to an array of new, satisfying and healthy food experiences.

---

108 E. Rosenbaum, et al., "Maintaining Good Nutrition," in *Everyone's Guide to Cancer*, 193.

CHAPTER 15

THINKING OUTSIDE THE BOX: ALTERNATIVE MEDICINE AND HOLISTIC APPROACHES

"Ideas are like rabbits. You get a couple and learn how to handle them and pretty soon you have a dozen."
John Steinbeck

For many people, a conventional, allopathic approach to treating cancer—one that involves chemotherapy, radiation or surgery (or a combination of these)—is simply not the way, or not the exclusive way, they want to go about treating their disease. For many of these people, an alternative or complementary medicine approach, one that involves a holistic/naturalistic path, is the one they choose exclusively or combine with their conventional treatment.

In a nutshell, holistic medicine is an approach that considers the mind, body and spirit to be interconnected in healing. Holistic medicine practitioners therefore seek to treat all of these aspects in curing disease. It incorporates considerations regarding a person's physical, nutritional, environmental, emotional, social, spiritual and lifestyle values and needs to reach a cure. Alternative or complementary medicine approaches to cancer treatment often incorporate these and other considerations.

Keep Your Heart and Eyes Wide Open

There are various types of alternative/complementary treatments that have gained some momentum or notoriety over the years, and many hospitals even make certain types of these treatments available in conjunction with conventional, allopathic cancer treatments. The proponents of alternative cancer treatments note the poor success rate of conventional treatments for certain types of cancer —especially metastatic cancers—and the highly toxic nature of treatments like chemotherapy and radiation, which kill healthy cells as well as cancerous ones. While alternative medicine remains controversial, many doctors feel that any therapy that reduces the pain, stress or depression of their patients is a positive and valuable aspect of treatment as long as it does not compromise their health. Bear in mind, however, that even doctors who are open-minded to alternative or complementary cancer treatments consider them to be ancillary to, and not a replacement for, conventional treatments.

Alternative or complementary medicine approaches, which often are not sanctioned or approved by governmental bodies tasked with regulating cancer treatments, include, among others, the following:

- Meditation/visualization: Meditative techniques, including helpful visualization (discussed elsewhere in this book), have been demonstrated in certain studies to reduce pain associated with cancer and its treatments and have been associated with an increase in the number of killer cells in cancer patients.[109] Meditation techniques have been associated with decreased anxiety and cortisol (stress hormone) levels, and some studies—but by no means all the studies that have investigated the issue—suggest that

---

109 See D. Podolsky, "New Acceptance of Alternative Cancer Treatments," in *Contemporary Issues*, 125.

meditation may improve the chance of a positive cancer outcome.[110]

- Nutrition: There are many people who have sought to cure their cancers through proper, professionally guided nutrition, and who survived despite eschewing conventional treatment. When I was at HHI and since that time I met several people who took this approach. Some had been treated conventionally but unsuccessfully, some used a nutritional approach in conjunction with conventional treatment and some chose to forego conventional treatments entirely. The monthly HHI newsletter, *Healing Our World*, almost invariably includes anecdotal stories of people who are convinced that adopting proper nutrition and a healthy lifestyle helped cure their cancer. As discussed in chapter 14, nutrition may play a role in the development, treatment and defeat of cancer. Explore nutritional approaches with your doctor and a qualified nutritionist, follow the basic guidelines set forth in chapter 14 and consult the more detailed sources referenced in that chapter. Make sure that any nutritional approach to curing cancer that may be recommended to you does not ignore or deprive you of critical nutrients your body will need to fight your cancer and heal. As a general rule, any diet that advocates *completely* foregoing entire nutritional areas should be avoided or, at a minimum, should be viewed with extreme caution (for example, although processed sugars and carbohydrates should be avoided, cutting out *all* carbohydrates or *all* sugars, even natural ones, can deprive the body of essential nutrients). There is no one "miracle" diet, although there are sensible ones rooted in natural, unprocessed foods that support your immune system, reduce inflammation, help lessen some

---

110 *Complete Guide*, 105–107.

of the difficult side effects of conventional treatments and promote healing.

- Immune-based therapies: There are several cancer therapies that are based on boosting the immune system. Dr. Gorter's approach is one of these. These therapies focus on building up and increasing the number and effectiveness of immune cells, including NK (killer) cells. Building up and reactivating a suppressed immune system certainly may help you heal. Again, however, some of these therapies may not have been subjected to extensive clinical testing or review, and the proponents of them, as with other alternative treatments, may have a financial interest in your following their program. Ask to see the data for such treatments and review them with your doctors to see if the immune therapy you are considering is for you.

- Detoxification and metabolic treatments: Another approach to treating cancer focuses on detoxification: ridding the body of toxins that have accumulated over the years, either through improper diet, environmental exposures, smoking or other poor lifestyle choices. The basic rationale underlying these approaches is that the body's natural inclination is to heal itself, but that things to which we are exposed or consume offset our biological balance and block the body's ability to heal. These metabolic approaches may include, in various degrees, diet, vitamin/mineral supplements, enzymes, sauna treatments and lymphatic and other types of massage and cleansing, including colon cleanses. To the extent that these approaches put you on the right path to nutrition, balance any vitamin or mineral deficiencies you may have and promote a sense of well-being, they can be very useful in helping you defeat your cancer. Treatments involved in some, but not all, of these approaches (including, for example, the injection of animal cells or consuming raw meat or raw meat juices) can be dangerous, however. While there is anecdotal evidence supporting their use for curing cancer, whether they in fact do so is a subject of considerable debate and, as with all alternative treatments, they should be reviewed with your doctor.[111]

- Hyperthermia: Hyperthermia is an approach in which tumorigenic tissues or areas of the body in which tumors are located are exposed to high temperatures (up to 113 degrees Fahrenheit or 40 to 43 degrees Celsius) to help destroy cancer cells. It has its roots in the Hippocratic idea that fever (i.e., elevated temperature) helps to cure disease. As Hippocrates said: "Those who cannot be cured by surgery can be cured by fire [hyperthermia]." Hyperthermia, which is often used in conjunction with conventional treatments, may make such treatments more effective by making cancer cells more susceptible to the effects of radiation or drugs.[112] Several studies have associated the inclusion of hyperthermia in cancer treatment with improvement in control of tumor spread and survival.[113] One such study noted that, with hyperthermia: "Significant improvement in clinical outcome has been demonstrated for tumors of the head and neck, breast,

---

111 See the American Cancer Society's review of metabolic treatments at http://www.cancer.org/Treatment/TreatmentsandSideEffects/ ComplementaryandAlternativeMedicine/DietandNutrition/ metabolic-therapy. See also Complete Guide, 646–650.

112 See, e.g., G. DeNardo and S. DeNardo, "Turning the Heat on Cancer," *Cancer Biotherapy and Radiopharmaceuticals*, vol. 23, no. 6 (2008): 671–680 at 671; B. Hildebrandt, et al., "The Cellular and Molecular Basis for Hyperthermia," *Critical Review Oncology/Hematology* (July 2002): 43(1):33–56.

113 See, for example, P. Wust, et al., "Hyperthermia in Combined Treatment of Cancer," *Lancet Oncology* (August 2002): 3(8):487–497.

brain, bladder, cervix, rectum, lung, esophagus, vulva and vagina, and also for melanoma."[114]

- Prayer: While most cancer patients, even devoutly religious ones, will not choose to leave their fate entirely in God's hands, to the exclusion of medical treatment, many will use the power of prayer as an aspect of their treatment therapy (and some, based either on their particular religious beliefs or aversion to conventional treatments, may choose to rely more heavily or even exclusively on prayer or faith healing techniques). As discussed in chapter 16, there are several studies showing a beneficial effect in terms of healing from religious faith and prayers. Whether such faith can fully "cure" cancer is controversial and is a personal issue that every cancer patient must answer for themselves.

While it is perfectly understandable for a cancer patient to seek out and cling to treatments that promise miraculous results without having to undergo the onerous conventional cancer treatments (chemotherapy, radiation and surgery), a healthy dose of caution is appropriate. Over the years, many alternative approaches that have been promoted for cancer treatment have arrived on the scene with much sound, fury and alleged promise, only to ultimately be relegated to the waste bin of useless cancer treatments. As with almost all things, if a recommended alternative treatment for your cancer seems "too good to be true," it probably is. Beware of people promoting "miracle cures," especially if they have a vested monetary interest in your following their method (if, for example, they own the product they are selling or are heavily invested in it, or are directing you to a clinic from which they derive substantial revenue). Although there are many alternative or complementary treatment approaches

---

114 J. van de Zee, "Heating the Patient: A Promising Approach?" *Ann Oncology* (August 2002): 13(8):1173–1184.

that may have merit and promise, there are, unfortunately, still many "snake oil salesmen" out there who will prey on vulnerable cancer patients while offering no real benefits.

That is not to say that such treatments or clinics should be rejected outright. For example, some years after my leukemia, when I was recovering from an attack of Stevens-Johnson Syndrome, I was searching online for the "best places to detox," and came across the website for HHI. Serendipitously, as I was reviewing the HHI website, a good friend called to see how I was feeling and told me that I should check out a place to which she had gone to treat her chronic fatigue. That place was HHI. Now, HHI is expensive and the people who run it make what I assume is a handsome profit from people going there, following their program and buying their supplements. They advocate a healthy, raw vegan diet, the use of wheatgrass, as well as exercise and stress relief, however. I went, and it changed my lifestyle for the better. I undertook a vegan diet, started using an infrared sauna on a near-daily basis to help me relax and rid my body of toxins and altered other aspects of my lifestyle.

The mere fact that the people at HHI had an interest in me attending and following their program did not for me derogate from the benefits of following that program. I met many other people there, including many cancer patients, who, having gone through the rigors of conventional cancer treatments, simply had decided that that route was no longer for them. Instead, they chose a holistic approach that focused on diet, exercise, detoxification, emotional support and stress relief. I even met a chemotherapy nurse there who had been diagnosed with stomach cancer. Having seen and administered chemotherapy to countless cancer patients, and having witnessed its effects over and over, she resolved not to go through that routine herself. While I do not know the long-term results for the people I met at HHI, many of them certainly began to look and feel better as they adopted the alternative approach promoted at HHI. The combined dietary/stress relief/meditation/exercise regimen offered by HHI and other clinics like it in all likelihood triggered some of the healthy reactions attendant to eliminating inflammatory foods and reducing stress.

At the same time, even at a place as established and popular as HHI, I encountered some positions that I disagreed with. One lecturer stated outright that "chemotherapy doesn't cure anyone." Although for many people chemotherapy either does not work or merely serves to lengthen—rather than improve—their lives, I felt that that representation went too far. There almost certainly were various elements involved in my survival, including my mental state and the support of my loved ones, but I also feel strongly that the chemotherapy regimen I went through played a critical role, and there are probably millions of people alive today who would not be if not for chemotherapy or radiation treatments. So even with regard to a place from which I and others benefitted tremendously, there were aspects of their philosophy with which I disagreed.

Vetting Complementary Treatments

In general, apply the same rigorous analysis and investigation to any alternative treatment that you would apply in considering a conventional treatment. Question and challenge anyone recommending such a treatment to you:

- Are there independent scientific studies supporting the efficacy of the treatment she is proposing? Peer review (review of scientific studies by the relevant scientific community) is the normal process by which treatments are evaluated. Most Western-trained physicians rely heavily on the scientific method of repeated, reliable studies subjected to peer review and comment as the basis for their approach to treating disease. One caveat, however, is that epidemiological studies (studies on human populations) cost hundreds of thousands, if not millions, of dollars and take years to perform. Even animal studies can cost substantial amounts of money to conduct. As a result, many such studies are funded by corporations (for example, pharmaceutical or chemical companies) that have a financial interest in promoting a certain type of drug or treatment or in at least understanding whether and how that drug or treatment works. There is often little money to be made by these corporations from alternative cancer treatments, several of which are readily accessible, inexpensive and possibly cannot be patented. Therefore, there may simply not be enough interest or money in performing the number and types of studies that many doctors and other scientists would want to see before recommending an alternative cancer treatment. If this is the case, your doctor should be able to get a hold of "case studies" (studies following the treatment of individual patients) and make an analysis of the potential strengths or dangers of an alternative treatment.

- Does the person promoting it have a financial interest in it? If so, be wary.

- Does the treatment require that you abandon other treatments? Did patients who used this treatment successfully use it exclusively or in conjunction with conventional treatments? Bear in mind that there are ramifications from abruptly stopping any treatment you may already be using.

- Are there potential side effects or detrimental effects from the proposed treatment? If so, what are they? Along the same lines, you must determine whether any suggested supplements called for by the alternative approach (vitamin or mineral) are contraindicated by medications you are taking or can cause side effects that may be particularly troubling for cancer patients. For example, can they cause an allergic reaction that would cause rashes or sores that will cause extreme discomfort or perhaps make you more susceptible to infection?

- Is the person who runs or is promoting the alternative treatment you are considering willing to speak directly to your oncologist about it? If not, that is another red flag.

Your consideration of alternative treatments may also encounter some resistance from your oncologist, particularly if you are considering an alternative approach that precludes conventional cancer treatments. There are several potential reasons for this reluctance. First, you are his patient. Your doctor feels an obligation to guide you to the course of treatment with which he or she is most familiar, confident and experienced. Bear in mind also that many Western-trained doctors have not been schooled in therapies beyond the allopathic regimens taught in medical school or utilized in their specialties. Moreover, as discussed above, many alternative treatments have not been subjected to the rigorous review process most doctors insist upon to determine a treatment's effectiveness. As a result, many doctors may be resistant to something that is outside their box.

Another issue at play in this resistance is exposure to liability. In today's litigious environment, doctors are particularly wary of giving any advice or advocating any treatment that does not have a substantial, scientifically proven basis, because they may expose themselves to malpractice lawsuits if the alternative treatment either does not work or exacerbates a condition. Many good oncologists are open-minded, however, when it comes to complementary approaches, including nutritional approaches and stress management techniques, especially if they are to be used in conjunction with conventional treatment. If your oncologist is not open-minded and you truly want to pursue an alternative treatment, seek out other opinions and discuss them with your treating physician. If she is resistant, ask her specifically why she rejects those alternatives.

Further, although most doctors (and cancer specialists in particular) try to stay up to date on the latest advances in cancer treatment, they get dozens of journals and newsletters relevant to their field. It is virtually impossible for them to keep abreast of every development that may be relevant to your treatment. Thus, they may simply be unaware of a particular alternative approach or the evidence that supports its use. Bring such sources to their attention and discuss them.

In many instances, alternative approaches invoke the maxim that "what is old is new again." Scientists are rediscovering nutritional approaches to treating cancer and "country doctor remedies" that our forefathers used to fight disease. In my own case, part of my treatment involved IV arsenic trioxide. Arsenic was used years ago to treat leukemia but fell into disuse when modern chemotherapeutic drugs were developed. I have little doubt that many doctors would have derided its use to treat leukemia as "archaic" or "quackery" in the years before my treatment. In parts of rural China and other parts of the world that did not have access to those modern chemotherapeutic drugs, however, doctors were experiencing success in treating leukemia patients with a concoction that included arsenic. As a result, a study was undertaken, in which I participated, in which arsenic trioxide was added into the regimen. The success associated with its use has resulted in it now being made part of the regular treatment plan for APL.[115]

---

115 See *Complete Guide*, 46.

Whether foregoing a conventional treatment approach is the right thing for you is something you should discuss with your doctor and knowledgeable alternative medicine practitioners and cancer nutritionists. The bottom line, again, is what is best *for you.* While your doctor may have strong feelings about (and opposition to) an alternative cancer treatment, if you feel after extensive investigation, research and consultation with your doctors and others that an alternative plan is best for you, do not be bullied into foregoing it. Remember that your mind is like a parachute: it only works when it is open.[116]

---

116 One resource to consult in searching for alternative treatments is the National Cancer Institute's Office of Cancer Complementary and Alternative Medicine (http://www.cancer.gov/cam/), which has been tasked with evaluating alternative approaches to cancer treatment. A comprehensive review of alternative/complementary cancer treatments also can be found in the *Complete Guide, supra.* Another informative source is Memorial Sloan-Kettering Cancer Center's integrative medicine site, www.mskcc.org/cancer-care/integrative-medicine. For a critical review of several alternative cancer treatment approaches, see Barrett, *supra.*

CHAPTER 16

FIND YOUR SOUL

"The greatest mistake in the treatment of diseases is that there are physicians for the body and physicians for the soul, although the two cannot be separated."

Plato

For many people who are diagnosed with or being treated for cancer, such time is the right time to turn to, or rediscover, their spirituality, whether rooted in their belief in God or a higher power of some other sort. Great comfort can be derived from finding or rediscovering your "soul" during this difficult time.

The actual curative role of faith is an issue of debate in the scientific community. However, the Office of Technology Assessment reported that a survey of articles published in the *Journal of Family Practice* over ten years found that 83 percent of studies on religiosity found a positive effect on physical health.[117] Some research has found that religious groups with orthodox beliefs and behavior have lower cancer death

---

117 American Cancer Society, "Spirituality and Prayer" at http://www.cancer.org/Treatment/TreatmentsandSideEffects/Complementaryan-dAlternativeMedicine/MindBodyandSpirit/spirituality-and-prayer ("Spirituality and Prayer").

rates.[118] Other studies have found no evidence of increased cure rates among religious, disease-stricken patients. If there are such positive curative effects, they may be due to the stress-relieving aspects of faith and the attendant enhanced immune function and production of killer cells as a result. There is more evidence for the ameliorative effects of spiritual involvement among cancer patients, as religious practices have tended to result in a better ability to handle treatment and disease-related pain.[119]

In my own case, I came into my cancer already a religious person. I prayed daily. I observed the rules of an orthodox Jewish life. I already had a relationship with God that could form the basis of my soul searching. In truth, other than fleeting moments of uncertainty and fear, I never really doubted my ability to defeat and survive my cancer. I saw very clearly most of the time that I would get better, and my spiritual beliefs gave me some of that fortitude. I made sure to keep up my rituals even in the hospital. I would ask, when necessary, to have my IV removed so that I could don the religious articles used in Jewish morning prayers (which are wrapped on the arm and placed on the head). I studied rabbinical works dealing with faith and recovery. I even wrote and had someone else deliver for me a sermon in synagogue on one of the Sabbaths during which I was in the hospital.

Still, even for a person who already is somewhat forearmed against cancer by his religious beliefs and faith in God, cancer can be a challenge. For some people, it can rattle those beliefs

---

118 See J. Dwyer, et al., "The Effect of Religious Concentration and Affiliation on County Cancer Mortality Rates," *Journal of Health and Social Behavior* (1990) 31(2): 185–202 (the authors concluded that their study suggested that religious beliefs and practices had a significant effect on malignancies of all types, digestive cancers and respiratory cancer); "Spirituality and Prayer."

119 Ibid.

and call into question the reward of faith. You may ask yourself, "I have been a loyal servant to God all these years, why is He punishing me with cancer? What have I done wrong?" The answer, of course, is nothing. Just because you have cancer does not mean that you are being "punished" for anything. As I discussed in chapter 2, the fact is that even righteous people are met with challenges and trials. If you believe in God, then you also probably understand that His plan is often concealed from us. Cancer can simply be God's way of making us stronger and giving us the appreciation for all life offers that is too often lost in the hustle and bustle of life.

If, however, believing that cancer is a "punishment" from God for a life gone awry leads you to a direction that improves your life or rectifies the "wrongs" you believe you have committed, there is no ultimate harm there. To the contrary, a belief that your life's path has been corrected—that you have been reset on your appropriate course—can itself be encouraging and aid in your emotional well-being and, thereby, your healing process.

To the extent that my own faith went through any challenges during my cancer ordeal, those thoughts were laid to rest conclusively by a visit I had with a "Kabbalist" rabbi (a practitioner of Jewish mysticism) immediately after I got out of the hospital following my initial round of high-dose chemotherapy.[120] The rabbi was visiting New York from Israel, and I met him and his son in a hotel in New York. When I entered the room, I was greeted by an elderly man with a long, white beard and a long, white robe. As soon as I walked into the room, he said to me, in Hebrew, "You have a problem with your blood."

---

120 Kabbalah, as an area of study and practice, has been around for centuries. The kind of study and practice among rabbis renowned for their mystic abilities is not the contemporary Kabbalah that has become a fad for certain entertainment personalities.

Now, I had not had any experience with a Kabbalist before, although I knew many respectable people who swore by the ability of certain people to "see" things, so I was very taken aback by his comment, as I had not told him or his son anything about my condition before I met them. Of course, since I was newly bald, it would not have been a great leap to conclude that I had some type of cancer, but at the same time his identification of the specific source of my cancer (my blood) impressed me. Before I sat down, he also said to me, "You have a scar on your knee from sports." I do, indeed, have a big scar on my right knee from an old basketball injury. I proceeded to sit down across from him and he went on, "Your father had a problem with his heart and your mother with her head." My father had had a triple bypass and my mother had had a brain tumor removed a couple of years prior. Then, among other things, he told me the names of my two daughters and told me that I was supposed to have more children, but instead God had given me a longer life. He advised me regarding some things to do on a spiritual level to aid in my healing and continued progress.

My meeting with the rabbi had a profound effect on me. His insights and knowledge about my condition and my family—without any previous information on these issues—was piercing. This was no television psychic experience. It gave me a newfound respect for things that occur on the spiritual plain that may simply be beyond our understanding, but it also reassured me that there was a bigger "plan" for me and that it stretched well beyond my having cancer. In other words, it gave me encouragement that I would survive and motivated me to be more than just someone who lived through cancer.

For other people who may not be religious, or even believe in God, there is nonetheless an avenue to be "spiritual." Even absent a connection to the "divine," it is possible to find your connection to others and your role—or potential role—in the world around you. That realization may come from some of the techniques laid out elsewhere in this book (meditation, visualization and forgiveness). For many people (myself included), spirituality can come from a sense of place. There may be a particular place that makes you feel calm and centered. It may help you focus and see your role in your family, your community, your country or even your planet. Identifying your spiritual place can be very helpful in restoring and centering your "soul."

Cancer has a humbling effect. It can make you realize your vulnerability and your need to rely on others. For many people in today's society, vulnerability and anything other than complete self-reliance are considered weaknesses to be avoided and hidden. Recognizing or being reminded that you are interconnected with others is not a bad thing, however. To the contrary, the feeling that you rely on others and they rely on you reinforces the (correct) impression that there are things that are bigger than ourselves, and that we must act to further the interests not only of ourselves but of others around us and our community. Having and being treated for cancer instructs us in humility. The perspective gained through it can flow into other areas of life, helping us to control our anger or give more thought to what we do and say. It gives us the chance to implement lessons we have learned through trial. *That* is spirituality.

Becoming more spiritual also helps in achieving acceptance of what you are going through. Reclaiming your center through spiritual exercises can lead you to a point where you can say without trepidation, "I have cancer. It is not insurmountable. There are many worse things that could be happening to me; things that could not be fixed or cured. I am fortunate and will focus on my fortunes and not my troubles." Coming to this point will improve your mood and reduce your fears. As someone once said, "Feed your faith and your fears will starve to death."

CHAPTER 17

THE THREE "P'S" OF SURVIVAL

*"Nothing in the world can take the place of persistence …
Persistence and determination alone are omnipotent."*
Calvin Coolidge

My cancer was a blessing. That seems like blasphemy to someone enduring it, I know. How can facing a potentially terminal disease, going through chemotherapy or other onerous treatments that make you feel sicker than you ever imagined, losing your hair and worrying about what will happen to you and your family be a blessing? Nonetheless, when viewed properly, cancer can in fact be a blessing—even if it is a blessing that is realized only through trials—particularly in terms of perspective gained and the appreciation for life that cancer brings.

Indeed, life's blessings are often only realized through the prism of challenges and difficulties. My father worked for years for the Port Authority of New York and New Jersey. A loyal, dedicated and conscientious worker, he moved up to a managerial level, only to be "early retired" some years before he planned to, in fact, retire willingly. I know that he was dismayed at the time, and probably felt that he was unappreciated and prematurely "put out to pasture," and he struggled with those feelings. A few years later, terrorists flew two planes into the buildings in which he worked, the World Trade Center. Had he not been given early retirement, who knows whether he would be alive today to have experienced his grandchildren and his continued marriage to my mother (now in excess of fifty years). Your cancer can bring you to the same type of realization, by focusing on what I call "the three P's": persistence, perspective and priorities.

Persistence

Chinese philosopher and educator Kongfuzi said: "In the battle between the river and the rock, the river will always win. Not through strength, but through persistence." Think about that. On the one hand, you have a hard stone; heavy, dense, seemingly unyielding and immovable. On the other hand, you have water: soft, malleable, constantly changing its shape to accommodate its constraints and surroundings. Yet, as Kongfuzi noted, the latter *always* prevails in the end over the former. Even if it is not immediately overwhelming, given enough time, persistence and force, sooner or later that water will wear away the much harder stone and create its own path. Water also is the ultimate adapter. In a square container water is square. In a round one it is round. It is for these reasons that famed martial artist Bruce Lee advised his students to be like water. Lee wanted his students to be able to adapt their fighting techniques to whatever situation they were in. You too may feel that you are too soft to overcome the stone-like obstacle that cancer appears to be. With sufficient persistence and adaptation to your situation, however, you can wear away that stone and ultimately overcome it and create your path to health.

Oftentimes what defeats—or even kills—a person is simply succumbing to defeat; allowing yourself to believe that you can take no more, that there is nothing more that can be done. We rationalize this reconciliation. We tell ourselves that something is just "too hard," that it is "more than we can take." We tell ourselves "rational lies." That is understandable. Sometimes things *do* seem too hard to accomplish. The first time you try to run a marathon, you may believe that it is impossible. After you have *done* it, however, you realize that it only *seemed* impossible. There are times when going through cancer and the treatment for it can bring us to a point where we want to say "no more," or "I can't do it." Most of the time, you *can* do it, and telling yourself that you cannot, a "rational lie," is dangerous and counterproductive.

Mr. Goldberg used to sit near me on Saturdays in synagogue. He was a survivor of Auschwitz. He lost his wife, his children and nearly his soul. He related to me a story of something that happened to him in the death camp that has stayed with and inspired me over the years. He said that, beaten down, nearly starved, with everything that was of value stolen away from him, he came to a point where he could take no more. He sat down where he was and said to himself, "If they want my soul, let them come and take it from me right here." Considering what he went through and where he was, no one could have blamed him for giving up.

Then someone said to him, "You can't stay here; it's not safe," and helped lift him up and escort him to another area. The area where he had collapsed was along the line that led to the infamous Dr. Mengele, to the devil's door itself. When he finally was seated elsewhere he said that he opened his eyes to see the person who had forced him up and onward, only to see that there was no one there. He felt convinced that an angel of God Himself had come to save him. But whatever that force was—be it human or supernatural—it moved him from death's door back to life, and he resolved to live. He did, in fact, live many more years, to a ripe old age, and raised a new family in America. *He persisted.* He survived. He thrived despite the seeming impossibility of doing so.

It may sound like a clichéd science fiction movie line, but every person battling cancer must, at some point, find his "force." Elsewhere in this book I have discussed the importance of finding your "why" to fight your cancer. You need to identify and keep in mind whatever it is that makes you push further when there is no more strength, whether it is a promise made to a loved one not to die, a vow made to yourself that you *will* see the milestones of your loved ones or the sheer, unmitigated anger at the beast inside you to which you refuse to acknowledge defeat. *Find your force. Be persistent.* As Winston Churchill implored Britons confronting an implacable enemy:

> This is the lesson: never give in, never give in, never, never, never, never—in nothing, great or small, large or petty—never give in except to convictions of honor and good sense. Never yield to force; never yield to the apparently overwhelming might of the enemy.

Cancer is no less than your enemy in a personal war. As long as there is any reasonable hope of defeating it, never surrender, even when that enemy seems overwhelmingly mighty. Never give in to it. Your persistence in fighting your cancer will teach you about the true extent of your capabilities and extend the terrain of your life beyond what you thought were the borders of your fortitude. *That is a blessing.*

Perspective and Priorities

Perspective and priorities go hand in hand, because cancer gives you both. They are the bright side to cancer and its treatments. That there is such a bright side may be hard to believe, especially if you are in the throes of treatment and enduring some of its difficult side effects. But these treatments, like cancer itself, clarify things. They too are a blessing.

I remember someone asking me when I first came out of the hospital after a month's stay what I appreciated most about being out. "Being able to urinate directly into a toilet without having to worry about collecting everything that comes out," I said. It was simple. It was perhaps too frank. But it was absolutely true. The simple pleasure of going to the bathroom normally was my most basic, clearest satisfaction. After my hospitalization, I also could go outside. I could stand in the sun. I could smell something other than the antiseptic odors of a hospital ward or the stench of illness coming from my hospital bathroom. I could move around without being tethered to an IV pole. I could shower without having to cover my IV port with plastic and not worry about the hot water running too long over certain parts of my body. I could change my clothes without having to first call a nurse for assistance.

Chemotherapy and other cancer treatments can bring such realizations home to you. They can make you grateful for the simplest things and clear your vision, so that these basic joys are appreciated as fully as they should be. Going through these ordeals, or other cancer treatments, can make you appreciate just how valuable it is to have a body that functions as it should.

I will never forget an incident that happened early in my courtship of my wife. She saw that when I came out of the bathroom I was muttering a blessing that involves giving thanks to God for a healthy excretory system. My wife, who was not raised in a religious home, said, "Don't tell me there's a blessing for going to the bathroom too."

"Imagine," I told her, "what it would be like if you couldn't go? Doesn't it make sense that we should be thankful that we can?" Not many of the things cancer can do are positive, but helping you see things clearly and prioritize them correctly is one of them.

In addition to making you appreciate things you may have taken for granted previously, having cancer and dealing with its remedy will focus you on what is truly important in life. Too often we succumb to a routine that is focused on what is truly unimportant in the larger scheme. If you asked one hundred people which is more important, their jobs or their families, all one hundred likely would say that their families are more important. Yet how much time does the average person spend working versus time spent enjoying their families? What does that say about where our daily priorities really are focused? Cancer changes that. It makes you realize what is *really* precious. Being in my own bed, holding my children, making love to my wife, seeing my friends and even getting back to work all have taken on for me an inestimable value. If you are lucky, you will never again make your family or friends secondary to other things.

As but one simple example, during my cancer ordeal, after I had come home from the hospital, my wife and I made it a point never to answer the phone during dinner. Why? Because I realized that doing so suggested to my children that whoever might be calling, even if it was someone we did not even know, was more important than the time I was spending with them at that moment. In addition, whereas, before my cancer, I might have told them to "wait a minute" as I finished a sentence I was writing or a conversation I was having related to work, after cancer I would, whenever possible, tell others to "hold on" while I addressed whatever questions my children had or if they wanted to show me their latest Crayola masterpiece.

Perhaps Melissa Bank, author of, among other works, *The Girls' Guide to Hunting and Fishing*, put it best:

> During chemo, you're more tired than you've ever been. It's like a cloud passing over the sun, and suddenly you're out. You don't know how you'll answer the door when your groceries are delivered. But you also find that you're stronger than you've ever been. You're clear.

Your mortality is at optimal distance, not up so close that it obscures everything else, but close enough to give you depth perception. Previously, it has taken you weeks, months, or years to discover the meaning of an experience. Now it's instantaneous.[121]

That is the blessing that cancer gives you. Count it every day.

---

121 M. Bank, *The Girl's Guide to Hunting and Fishing*, 221.

PART IV

WHAT LIES WITHIN US
Navigating the Road Ahead

CHAPTER 18

DIG YOUR WELL BEFORE YOU NEED THE WATER

"The man who is prepared has his battle half fought."
Miguel de Cervantes

While I encourage you to maintain a positive frame of mind and to keep your sense of humor intact as you go through your cancer ordeal, there are certain things that you should take care of, if you have not already. This is not reconciling to defeat. Being prepared is not being fatalistic. It is being *realistic*. Planning (really the fourth "P") is not pessimism. It is practicality.

When There's a Will, There's a Way

If you do not already have a will, have one prepared. Many people simply put off this task until they feel like they have to do it, which is what happens when someone gets cancer. Every state has different rules regarding what a will should contain, how it needs to be executed and the forms that are acceptable. Forms for acceptable wills in most states can be found online, and you can save substantial legal fees by at least preparing a first draft by yourself. I would encourage you, though, to have your draft reviewed for completeness and enforceability by a lawyer in your home state. Set out specifically in your will how you want to devise your property. While big-ticket items (homes, cars and savings) may simply be bequeathed to your spouse or children, there may be specific items of personal property with sentimental value that you would want particular people to have. There is no personal property you own that cannot be left to someone.

You may also need to designate a particular guardian for your children if they are minors. This can be very difficult for any parent, as it requires you to envision your children growing up without you. Nonetheless, it must be done. Your spouse is the obvious first person to act as a custodian in your absence and by law most likely will have custody if anything happens to you. You should, however, still make provisions for custody of your children if, for whatever reason, your spouse becomes unable to care for them.

Who the best secondary guardians would be is a difficult, individualized decision that should involve your head as well as your heart. Grandparents are one choice, but bear in mind that, as people age—and their own children become independent and leave the home—their patience for small children, even their own grandchildren, on a constant basis may be limited. Moreover, placing your children full-time with aging grandparents may expose them to a situation where *they* will become caretakers if your parents themselves become infirm. In addition, these "replacement" parents are likely to pass away sooner than a younger custodian, forcing your children to again endure the loss of a parental figure.

Your siblings may also be good choices, but try as best you can to designate the best one for the job. Consider whether your siblings have the same overall values that you have tried to instill in your children. Do they have like-aged children (and do any of those children have behavioral or other issues that will affect your children or interfere with them getting the attention they will need)? Do they live very far away, such that your children will have to be uprooted and removed from all that is familiar to them? Do they have the financial wherewithal to provide for your children properly?

Another alternative is a close family friend, with whom you and your children have a deep bond. Ask the same questions listed above in making such a choice and discuss it with those friends before you designate them. As much as you may love your friends and they may love you, they simply may be unprepared to shoulder the responsibility of raising and caring for your children. Also, if you decide to go outside of your family for a custodian, explain to your family members why you are doing so. Failure to do so inevitably will result in hurt feelings, recriminations and, possibly, an ugly custody fight.

In addition, if you have particular desires for how you want to be treated after you pass away, put that in the will as well. Setting out your wishes in a will can (hopefully) preclude any bickering later on over what your intentions were. In recent years, many people have chosen to prepare recorded or videotaped wills. If you do this, check the laws of your state to make sure such a will is valid and what the requirements are for making one. Try to do it before the effects of your treatment are manifest. Let your family see you as they always remembered you. In your own words, give them your blessing and permission to go on with their lives and be happy. Tell them how much their love meant to you and that they should celebrate your life as opposed to mourning your death.

Make Arrangements

By the same token, make sure whatever needs to be done for a funeral is done. If you do not own a funeral plot, you may want to consider purchasing one (like a will, you will need it someday anyway, hopefully many years from now). You can describe in your will what type of funeral arrangements you would like to have.

Another practical arrangement you should consider is a power of attorney. If you are undergoing extensive and onerous cancer treatments or are very sick, or you are having surgery that requires general anesthesia, a power of attorney will give someone else the temporary power to make medical and legal decisions for you if you are incapacitated. Failure to have one in place can lead to bitter disagreements among your loved ones as to what the best approach to your treatment and care should be. Again, many state-specific forms for such a document can be found online, but run any drafts you prepare past an attorney to make sure it is done properly and is enforceable.

Similarly, you may want to consider and discuss with your doctor filling out a Do Not Resuscitate (DNR) order. This document directs hospital staff not to administer resuscitative treatment under certain circumstances (for example, administering CPR). *Bear in mind that DNR orders are generally only appropriate for people who are terminally ill and for whom continued treatment is either unlikely to help or who simply no longer wish to try to prolong their lives, when their suffering has become too great.*

It is not uncommon for one person in the family to handle certain matters, whether it is balancing the budget, paying the bills, keeping track of investments or staying on top of extracurricular activities. When that person gets sick, however, this routine can be thrown into disarray. All of a sudden things that used to get done may fall by the wayside, further upsetting a life already disturbed by cancer. Make sure your spouse or children know what they need to know: where the bank accounts are (and the account numbers); who handles your life insurance and investments and how to contact that person; what the schedule is for hockey practice or dance recitals and who else drives the carpool. This will make your transition into "fighting cancer" mode go more smoothly.

CHAPTER 19

IF THE END BECOMES INEVITABLE

*"And in the end, it's not the years in your life
that count. It's the life in your years."*

Abraham Lincoln

For some cancer patients, the best treatments, greatest attitude, most open mind and most loving support system will not prevent the disease from progressing and, ultimately, taking their life. Although, as time goes on, advances in cancer treatment save people—like me—whose cancers previously were not survivable, the harsh fact remains that despite these advances and the strongest, most positive attitudes and hopes, some cancer patients die. The incomparable comedienne, Gilda Radner, who fought her own courageous battle against, and ultimately succumbed to, cancer, wrote in her book, *It's Always Something*:

> I wanted a perfect ending. Now I've learned, the hard way, that some poems don't rhyme, and some stories don't have a clear beginning, middle, and end. Life is about not knowing, having to change, taking the moment and making the best of it, without knowing what's going to happen next.

If you find yourself in a situation where death becomes a near certainty, there are still things within your power to do that can affect what time you have left and *how* you die. You can still, as Gilda Radner said, take the moments that remain and make the best of them. What matters is that, during your life, you have *lived*.

That you may not achieve everything you wanted to do does not matter. In truth, even if we all lived to be one hundred, there would still be work for us left undone. The fact is that we *never* complete the most important jobs in life: being a parent, child, spouse, sibling or friend. But, as the *Ethics of the Fathers*, a book of rabbinical wisdom, instructs, "It is not incumbent upon you to complete the work."[122] Rather, each generation leaves undone some tasks for the next generation to achieve. Our legacies are like a puzzle, and each generation adds its own pieces to that puzzle. Even if you are unable to place as many pieces into the puzzle as you would like, what is most important is that the pieces you *do* insert guide those who come next to see the bigger picture and help them add *their* pieces. As Nelson Henderson wrote, "The true meaning of life is to plant trees, under whose shade you do not expect to sit."

"It's a good day to die" is a quote attributed to Thasunjke Witko, a Lakota Sioux holy man otherwise known as Crazy Horse, who is perhaps best known for leading the war party against General Custer at the Little Big Horn. It reflects his reconciliation with the possibility of death. It indicates his recognition that his life was well lived, and that the battle he faced was worth fighting, worth fighting well and, if necessary, that his cause was worth dying for. It shows a man at peace with his accomplishments and how he would be remembered. That same reconciliation was expressed centuries ago: "I have fought a good fight, I have finished my course, I have kept the faith."[123] You too ultimately can

---

122 *Ethics of the Fathers*, 2:21.
123 2 Timothy 4:7.

decide that it is a "good day to die," if you can reconcile yourself to a life well lived and make the path toward the end your own. Dying from cancer does not have to mean that you have been *defined* or *defeated* by it.

Once you have reached this point, all decisions regarding your path fall on you. Your doctor can guide you toward treatments or drugs that may ease pain or even prolong your life to a certain extent. Whether to adopt these approaches, however, is something you will have to decide. You may choose to undergo any and every treatment available, even the most aggressive or unproven, in order to stretch out your life as long as possible or achieve a miracle (and, as discussed elsewhere in this book, they sometimes do happen). For some people, the most important thing is squeezing as much time out with loved ones as possible. Others cling tenaciously to life to reach a milestone or because they hope for a last-minute cure. Still other people continue their fight to the very end because they want to delay the grief their family and friends will suffer when they pass away. There is certainly nothing wrong with any of these approaches, provided they are *your* decision. But bear in mind that you may continue to deteriorate, experience increased pain and put your loved ones through the additional trauma of seeing your life and energy ebb away.

On the other end of the spectrum are people who, faced with the inevitability of death, choose to stop fighting and putting their body through the difficulty of cancer treatments. In the alternative, they may continue their treatments or modify them to be directed toward pain management or providing as much quality of life as possible in the remaining time. There is no shame in this approach either. If we are lucky in life, unlike someone who dies very suddenly, we may have the chance to, to a certain extent, choose *how* we die. If you choose to avoid the potential humiliation of seeing yourself weakened further or choose to forego treatments that are unlikely to help heal you in order to keep your family from watching you go through them, that is noble as well. And while your doctor's main job and focus have been to help you get well, all oncologists are versed in the reality that some patients die, and they can advise you as to how to lessen any remaining suffering as you live out the time you have left.

In the end, whether you die from cancer or from another cause late in life, as Shi Dejian, kung fu master and Shaolin monk, said, "You cannot defeat death; but you can defeat your fear of death."[124] We can also, to a certain extent, counter any feelings of impotency that may come in the face of death by asserting control over the things we *can* control and our attitude as the end of our physical lives comes nearer. Controlling, as much as possible, how your last days are spent is one way to help you do so.

You should endeavor to die in a way that will make an indelible, positive impression on those around you. There is, in fact, a way to "survive" even after your physical life ends. The impression we leave on those around us ensures a legacy that will have an impact for many years to come. Let your family and friends see your courage as well as your fears. Face the end with humor and spirit. Reminisce with those you love about the many good, happy times and experiences you have shared. Revisit the stories that made you laugh until it hurt. Remind yourself and others that your life has had great meaning.

You may choose to record messages or write letters to those you will leave behind, especially children, to be viewed at certain times in their lives (graduations, anniversaries, weddings or the birth of your grandchildren). Include in those messages how much you loved them and how proud you are of them, and that you wish them all the happiness that

---

124 "Shaolin Kung Fu," *National Geographic* (March 2011).

you had with them in life. Encourage them to find happiness even if you are not there in body to share that happiness with them.

Make your peace with yourself and, if you believe, with God. Make amends. Invariably, throughout each of our lives, there are people who, intentionally or not, we have wronged, insulted, offended or made to feel bad. You may carry some guilt over these things. Fix that. Reach out to anyone who may fall into this category, apologize sincerely and make things right. As the sage Hillel advised, "If not now, when?"[125] Some of these people may reject your overtures of peace and others will welcome them and surprise you with their support. In any event, unburdening yourself and making sincere attempts to rectify any past wrongs can have a liberating effect on you and release your emotional energies. It may also simply help you reestablish friendships you wish you had never lost in the first place. In the same vein, *forgive.* Just as seeking forgiveness and making amends for your actions can unburden your soul, releasing others from the bonds of grievances or grudges you hold against *them* also releases negativity, can improve your own mood and will help reconcile you to your physical departure from this world.

Like most people, you probably have been a good person. You have brought value to those around you and have influenced them in a positive way. Whether you are conscious of it on a daily basis or not, you have made significant contributions to the world you encountered by sharing special relationships, helping others through your work (even if it was not your intention to do so) or encouraging other people to do their best. Following your example, the people you leave behind will honor your legacy by living up to the principles you taught them and encouraging future generations of your

---

125 *Ethics of the Fathers,* 1:14.

descendants or theirs—even those you will never know—to emulate them. Your example of courage and grace in the face of cancer will leave behind a wake of inspiration to others. When *their* lives are difficult in some way they will remember how you dealt with the hardships of cancer with bravery, humor and spirit, and will be strengthened by your example.

As Rabbi Wein wrote:

> What is the best way to be remembered? In a family situation, it is by the warmth and love exhibited to one's children and relatives. It is by the family dinners eaten together, with the computer turned off and the phone disconnected. It is by thoughtful, kind and positive conversation, by touching and soothing, by smiles and laughter and tears. ... My grandfather, whom I remember vividly though he died when I was just 10 left us no meaningful material wealth, but rather bequeathed to us a host of spiritual gifts and memories. And amazingly enough, my own grandchildren, generations later, when they pass his picture hanging in our home, seem to also 'remember' him because of shared moral and spiritual values and religious traditions which transcend time and generations, and which allow for positive and unending memory.[126]

So too the warmth and encouragement you have given to, the moral guideposts you have erected for and the values you have instilled in those around you will create a legacy that will long outlive your physical life.

I went to high school with Bruce. He was a young-looking, skinny kid. He was good natured and everyone liked him. When we graduated, he was given an award for outstanding personal qualities, and the entire class stood up and cheered when he got that award. Bruce and I lost touch

---

126 Wein, *Buy Green Bananas*, 188–189.

after high school, but many years later a mutual friend who had seen me through my leukemia told me that Bruce was battling lymphoma. I reached out to Bruce on Facebook and let him know that I had been where he was and I was always available to talk to him. We wound up reestablishing a long-lost relationship and counseling with each other through his battle.

Ultimately, after extensive treatment, Bruce had beaten his cancer. In addition to making me extremely happy for him and his family, it gave me great personal satisfaction when, having achieved remission, he wrote me that my encouragement and counsel had "helped [him] through some tough times this past year," and that he, in turn was "paying it forward" by counseling another cancer patient. So ready for the rest of his life was he that he and his family undertook a pilot trip to Israel to investigate the possibility of moving there. Tragically, on that trip, Bruce contracted double pneumonia. After the ravages of cancer and chemotherapy, his system simply was too weak to fight through it and he passed away.

I was devastated to hear of his passing, breaking into tears in my office upon getting the news. We had promised each other to celebrate our respective remission anniversaries together in the future. I find myself occasionally going back to his Facebook page, as if he might yet be posting messages. When I go back to our high school, I sometimes look at my class' graduation picture and linger on his image. I miss him. He was a friend and a comrade in arms.

But although Bruce died, he *survives*. Many of his friends and classmates repeated a common theme about the person he was: that none of us ever heard him say a bad word about anyone. How many people could have that comment made honestly about them? We all remembered his kindness and good nature. Even through the decades, his example continued to touch us. Shortly after his passing, his wife began soliciting stories from his friends and family that she could assemble for their young children so that they could have a remembrance of who their father was. Bruce's legacy of goodness, and the example he set for all those he touched, will be carried on by his children. *Bruce goes on.*

That can be true for you as well. The endeavors of *your* loved ones, how they live, love and teach *their* children, will reflect your qualities and their love for you. As Thomas Bailey Aldrich wrote: "What is lovely never dies, but passes into other loveliness."[127] Even after death, you will go on. You will survive.

---

127 T.B. Aldrich, *A Shadow of the Night.*

CHAPTER 20

FOR THOSE LEFT BEHIND

"What lies behind us and what lies before us are tiny things compared to what lies within us."

Ralph Waldo Emerson

When someone dies from cancer, the surviving family members and other loved ones can go through an enormous range of emotions. You may obviously feel the grief of loss. The person you loved will no longer in this life be there physically. Gone are the hugs, conversations, laughter and comfort of having that person around, and that is a huge loss. But ever present are the *memories* of hugs, conversations, secrets shared and comfort that person brought to you over the years.

Adults Left Behind

Many people internalize their grief and suffer with it silently. Strive not to do so. Just as a cancer patient can benefit tremendously from unburdening herself or sharing her feelings with someone she loves and trusts, a bereaved loved one also can benefit from doing so. Often it is not the grief alone that is so difficult to bear, but rather the erroneous feeling that it must be borne silently or alone. Indeed, certain religious rituals associated with death (for example, sitting shiva in the Jewish tradition or having a "viewing" or a wake, or even a memorial service) are designed so that the aggrieved family members do not have to endure the loss of their loved one alone. Find someone you trust and love and share your feelings with them. In the course of doing so, make a point of reliving the many positive events and feelings you associate with the person who has passed away. Laugh at the memories and relish all the gifts that that person gave you.

Other emotions also can come into play. Guilt is a prevalent emotion in these circumstances. A loved one often feels as if he simply "didn't do enough" or should have done or said something—or should have avoided doing or saying something—to help the patient or ease the patient's suffering. These feelings are almost always misguided. In all likelihood, you did everything you could for the person you loved. You visited, you called, you encouraged, you cooked, you prayed, you listened and you loved. Just as even the greatest doctors sometimes lose patients, the difficult fact is that sometimes the best we can do simply is not enough to get the results we want. There are sometimes things that are simply out of our hands. Most important, be honest with yourself. If your lost loved one was in front of you and could answer the question "Was there something more I should have done?" he or she would answer unequivocally, "No," and reassure you that your love and devotion through the course of their cancer sustained and helped them in ways you could never imagine. Sometimes, even if your best does not seem like enough to *you*, in actuality it is *more* than enough for the person you were trying to help.

After a loved one endures a long and arduous battle with cancer, another difficult feeling someone left behind may have is a sense of relief; a sensation of gladness that the person who was sick for so long—and who unintentionally placed a strain and burden on those around him—is gone. No more long days and nights in the hospital. No more having to bathe and dress and feed someone too weak to do so for herself. No more delaying a much-needed vacation because there was no one else to care for a sick person. Finally, it is over.

That feeling is not unusual. It comes, however, with the concomitant emotion of guilt. It may be impossible not to feel, on some level, a sense of relief when the burden of caring for a seriously ill cancer patient—and that burden can be both physically and emotionally exhausting—is lifted. *Forgive yourself* for that emotion. In all likelihood, the loved one for whom you were expending so much physical and emotional energy *regretted* your having to do so, and never wanted to be the burden they became. That person himself would feel relief at seeing *you* relieved of having to care for him. That you may feel relieved, therefore, is actually what your loved one would have wanted.

In addition, when a cancer patient passes away, the loved ones he or she leaves behind may feel incapable of happiness—or guilty about experiencing joy. It may seem inappropriate to laugh or love with another person. That too is a common feeling. We spend so much of our lives tied emotionally to the person who has left us that we feel like we are betraying her if we experience happiness in her absence. "How can I have fun when he is gone?" you may ask yourself. "How can I embrace another woman after having lived with and shared my love exclusively with her for so many years?" I believe that the answer lies in some advice I gave a grieving mother some years ago.

When I was at HHI, there was a young woman there from England named Mandy. Mandy recently had lost a child, and she was obviously and justifiably devastated. Her grief was preventing her from functioning and was having an adverse effect on her marriage. Her husband needed her to get past her grief so he could also feel better and they could begin to heal as a couple. He was frustrated and stressed over his inability to help her.

In a group session, I told Mandy to visualize her lost son in front of her. I asked her, "Mandy, if your son was here in front of you today, what do you think he would tell you? Don't you think he would say to you, 'Mommy, be happy. I don't want you to be sad?' Of course he would," I assured her, because the people we love and who love us want that more than anything. They want us to be happy, and the way we live our lives honors them only if it is the way they would have *wanted* us to live. Mandy told me afterward that she was committed to taking my words to heart and honoring her child by endeavoring to find happiness.

Your loved one would have wanted you to find a way to be happy even in her absence. Indeed, I have a friend who devotedly nursed his wife of many years through cancer until the very end of her life. Before she died, she not only encouraged him to remarry, but *told him who she had in mind for him.* (They are, in fact, now happily married.) Wallowing in grief or avoiding joy is exactly what she would *not* want for you, and you are betraying her memory by doing so. That is not to say that you are not allowed to grieve or that your grief will disappear even if you undertake these steps. But if you want to honor the memory of your loved one, find a way to be as happy as she would have wanted you to be.

This may not be easy for you. Doing things you enjoyed with the person who has passed away inevitably will involve some grief as you feel the loss most acutely in those circumstances. But the things you enjoyed previously will likely still bring you joy. If possible, find a friend with whom to do them. Express to your friends that it is still okay to include you in activities (they may feel awkward, not knowing what you are ready for, not wanting to bring you any sorrow or simply thinking erroneously that you no longer want to be included). In addition, take up new activities, especially ones that would have made your lost loved one proud. Try some of the things you always wanted to do but never took the time for. If that activity (a trip, learning to play an instrument, going back to school, etc.) is something you and your loved one hoped one day to do together, you will honor his memory by pursuing that dream.

Children Left Behind

Children, especially young children, of a patient who ultimately succumbs to cancer can be affected in profound ways, just as they can be affected when you are going through and being treated for cancer. They may become more introspective. They may start to act out or develop discipline problems as they deal with the loss of someone who has always provided a source of strength and stability for them. Their grades may drop off and they may show disinterest in activities they formerly enjoyed, especially activities they did with the parent or loved one who has passed away. Some children may experience or express a desire to die themselves, in order to reunite with their lost parent.

Children often see their parents as indestructible and come to rely on them as a constant in their lives; people to whom they can always go to make their problems or fears go away. Parents are a source of love, guidance and discipline. Children expect their parents to take care of them when they are sick, encourage them when they are down and protect them from things that are scary. More than anything, children expect their parents simply to *be there*.

Unlike adults who have developed their own personalities and have careers and other things to center them or help them reestablish a routine, and who may already have experienced the loss of someone close to them, such as a parent, children are not yet fully developed emotionally or intellectually. Therefore, when a parent is taken away suddenly they may feel as if all of their expectations for how life is supposed to be have unraveled. The loss of that person can rattle a child's sense of equilibrium and throw into disarray their previously held beliefs about life and their own security or even mortality.

In fact, research studies have shown that many children who experience the death of a parent manifest symptoms of anxiety, particularly regarding the potential for other family members to die, and that this anxiety can continue for several months, as a form of posttraumatic stress disorder. Symptoms include sleep disturbances,[128] strained peer relations and impaired school performance.[129] Some children go back to their usual routines after a short period of grief. That does not mean, however, that they have gotten over the loss. Children's emotions, like their bodies, are often more elastic than those of adults, and you need to keep your finger on the pulse of their reactions following a loss.

There are many things you can and should do to help your child cope with this devastating loss. You must reassure her that she is not alone, that there are still many people who love her and will watch over her. You should remind her of how much her parent loved her and how he or she will always be with her, even if she cannot see or talk to him directly.

---

128 Such sleep issues may relate to the association children make between sleep and death (as an unending type of sleep). See A. Sadeh, "Stress, Trauma and Sleep in Children," Child and Adolescent Psychiatric Clinics of North America (1996) 5(3):685–700. Considering that children are often told that someone who has died has "gone to sleep and won't wake up" and that death in other circumstances is compared to sleeping (for example, putting a pet "to sleep"), that a child might associate sleeping with dying is not surprising.

129 E. S. Harris, "Adolescent Bereavement Following the Death of a Parent: An Exploratory Study," Child Psychiatry Hum. Dev. (Summer 1991): 21(4):267–281.

Some years ago, a good friend of ours passed away suddenly at the age of thirty-seven, leaving behind several young children. Among the comments that one of his children made was that it was okay that Daddy had died because, "When he was alive, he worked so much that we hardly got to be with him. Now he is with us all the time."[130]

Listen to the questions your child asks and answer them sincerely and honestly. You should encourage her happy memories of the times spent with the parent she has lost. Do not shy away from talking about the lost parent. Indeed, studies have shown that a child's ability to deal effectively with grief following the loss of a parent is tied directly to the strength of the surviving parent's relationship with that child and the openness with which that parent addresses the death and the child's feelings about it, including talking about the deceased parent.[131]

Among the factors that have been shown to help children reconstitute their lives as much as possible after the loss of a parent include: (i) having a relationship with the surviving parent or caregiver characterized by open communication, warmth and positive experiences; (ii) having a competent surviving parent; (iii) feeling accepted by peers and other adults, including other relatives and teachers; and (iv) the opportunity to express thoughts and feelings about the deceased parent and have them validated by others.[132] If your child has difficulty speaking about the loss, encourage him

---

130 His wife, also a dear friend, ultimately remarried a man whose wife similarly had passed away at an early age, leaving him with several children. They went on to join their families together and, in fact, added to their new family. I have little doubt that that is what our friend would have wanted for his wife and children in his absence.

131 See "Helping Children Cope." This article contains an excellent compendium of issues that arise when a parent has or succumbs to cancer and how to address those issues.

132 Ibid.

to write a letter about how he feels, even a letter addressed to the parent who has died. Do not put away pictures to try to shield her from pain, as doing so will in all likelihood just reinforce the sense of loss and instability she feels.

Be sensitive when deciding what personal articles of your loved one's belongings to get rid of. Invite your child into the process and offer her particularly significant personal items that she can associate with her parent and the relationship she had with them. Children often have an attachment to clothing or other items that belonged to the deceased parent and they should not be alienated from those items. Once you have identified and set aside those personal items you and your children wish to keep, donate your loved one's things to charity and explain to your child that you are going to give away his parent's things to help other people, and that you want him to be involved in that project because that would make his parent proud.

As much as you may want to help your child heal from the loss of their parent, however, the fact is that most of us simply are not prepared to understand and address the full panoply of emotions that a child may experience when she loses a parent. Effective techniques for helping your child deal with that loss or express their emotions in a positive way are outside the lexicon of most laypeople. This is all the more difficult when you are dealing with your own sense of loss.

It is important for you to realize that you may not be prepared fully to help your child through this ordeal. Seek out professional help for your child. Do not assume that any significant changes in your child's behavior or attitude are a phase that will pass as the loss grows further into the distance. An uncorrected path may lead a child on a damaging journey from which recovery may be difficult if the path is not corrected quickly. Gone are the days when psychological counseling bore some sort of stigma. A school psychologist or your pediatrician may be good starting points, especially if she is someone your child knows and with whom he already has some sense of trust. She may also be able to refer you to someone with particular expertise in dealing with bereaved children. To the extent possible, interact with a therapist with your child so that you can understand what she is going through and how you can help.[133]

There is no simple or exclusive path to dealing with the loss of your loved one or helping others do so. Much of the path will seem unsure and uneven, but it is not uncharted. Many others have gone through the same experience as you and there are resources available to help you through it, in the form of counselors, friends and support groups. Your loved one's doctor or hospital may even be able to direct you to people who can help you and your family get through your loss. Take advantage of them and always keep in mind and be driven by the principle discussed above: that your loved one would have wanted more than anything else for you to be happy. Find a way to be so.

---

133 For suggestions regarding how to spot and deal with the effects of the loss of a parent on your child, see also "Helping Children when a Family Member has Cancer: When a Child has Lost a Parent" at http://www.cancer.org/Treatment/ChildrenandCancer/HelpingChildrenWhenaFamilyMemberHasCancer/WhenaChildHasLostaParent/index.

CHAPTER 21

LIFE-CHANGING EVENTS
SHOULD CHANGE YOUR LIFE

"Difficult times have helped me to understand better than before, how infinitely rich and beautiful life is in every way, and that so many things that one goes worrying about are of no importance whatsoever."
Karen Blixen (aka Isak Dinesen)

Many people have asked me whether my life has changed significantly since I went through my cancer battle. My answer to them has been that if you go through a life-changing event and your life does not change, you have a problem. Your life *should* be different as a result of being diagnosed with, going through treatment for and surviving your cancer. You are—or will be—a *survivor*. But there is a difference between *survival* and *recovery*. Although you have survived your cancer in the sense that you have lived through it and rid your body of it, you probably will never "recover" from it. Your cancer will be "part" of you long after it has been driven from your body. It may no longer be boiling on your front burner, but it may simmer somewhere on the back of your mental stove. And that is not necessarily a bad thing.

There certainly may be a lingering, potentially negative aspect of your cancer ordeal, in terms of your concerns about your health going forward. I can recall quite clearly a couple of experiences that happened during my consolidation treatments, when I was already technically in remission, which affected me profoundly. During my subsequent arsenic trioxide treatments, my daily blood counts had taken a dip. Understandably, I was scared. I did not know at the time whether this was a normal part of my recovery. I can recall very distinctly doing what a lot of people do in such circumstances—making a "deal" with God. If He would make those results just a blip on my way to wellness, I would be better in so many things. In fact, the kind of fluctuation I was experiencing was normal. I just did not know that at the time. The chemotherapy nurse reassured me that what I was experiencing was common and that I was probably fine. Still, I was not at peace until my next results showed an uptick in my cell counts.

At the beginning of another week of treatment, I went in as usual for my blood tests, and then proceeded to have my treatment. Later that afternoon, my doctor called me at home and asked me how I was feeling. When I asked him why, he told me that my blood test results from earlier that day were "unintelligible." When I asked him what he meant, he told me simply that the results "didn't make any sense," and that I would need to have the tests redone the next morning. Needless to say, I was a little panicked. Were my blood counts too low? Was my chemotherapy not working? Was I slipping out of remission? That night was long and sleepless.

The next day, I went back to the hospital to have my blood tests redone. I waited tensely in the waiting room for the results. Finally, after what seemed like hours (but was probably no more than thirty minutes), the doctor and one of the women running my protocol came out and started walking in my direction. My heart was pounding. "Here it comes," I thought, "my cancer is back." They told me, however, that my blood counts were fine; that the previous day's results probably were skewed by some of the Heparin, which had been used to flush my medi-port, getting into the blood sample. Almost immediately, I broke out into uncontrollable sobbing—one of those long, heaving sobs you experience when a flood of emotions rushes out of you. But even in the midst of my treatment, when my concerns were completely justified, in fact those concerns turned out to be unfounded.

You too may worry more over illnesses that would not have worried you before or stress over whether they mean that your cancer is returning. A common, lingering cold or cough, which you would have shrugged off previously, may concern you. A fever may cause you to worry in a way you would not have before your cancer. An inexplicable pain in your side or back or an unexplained bruise may keep you up at night for reasons wholly unrelated to the pain itself. That is normal. It may, in fact, be a type of posttraumatic stress from which many cancer survivors, me included, suffer. Relax. The illnesses you experience post-cancer are, in all likelihood, the same illnesses you experienced pre-cancer. They are likely the same common ailments most people get from time to time, and you probably will be fine.

That is not to say, however, that you should ignore something out of the ordinary. If you get sick and do not seem to get better, or feel extremely run-down, or become in some other way symptomatic of your prior cancer, follow up with your doctor immediately. Some cancers do return to fight another day, and you must make sure to beat them down as soon as they do. But try to remind yourself of the steps you have taken to defeat your cancer. You went through treatment. You endured months of feeling lousy to reach a cure. You kept your spirits up and your sense of humor intact. You changed your lifestyle for the better. You refused to be defeated. You did a lot and, in all likelihood, you beat it. A later illness is most likely unrelated to your cancer.

You may also experience a phenomenon of survivor's guilt. I have experienced it several times myself. Just as during your cancer you may ask "Why me?" the same question in a different light arises when you have survived. You may wonder why you have lived when others did not. This is especially so when someone you have come to know or is close to you dies from cancer.

I went through that emotion profoundly when my friend Bruce, whom I discussed in chapter 19, passed away. I have been able to go on with my life and he could not. I have seen my children grow and develop into beautiful young adults and have been able to enjoy them at a level he never had a chance to experience. They, in turn, have had the chance to know and learn from me in ways that Bruce's children never will. I have felt "guilty" about all of this, especially because I always believed him to be my moral superior. He was "better" than I am, and yet he died and I remain.

Although I only came to realize it fully years after my cancer battle, part of my "why," and part of the answer to "Why me?" lay in using my experiences to write this book. That epiphany only truly came to me when Bruce died. Like the solitary candle I discussed in chapter 11 that changes the look and feel of a dark room, or lights the way on an unclear path, the fact that I needed to reach out to as many other cancer patients as possible and help them and their families navigate through this bumpy road, as I tried to do with Bruce, was illuminated for me by his passing, and I recommitted myself to finishing this road map. I knew that I needed not only to live, but to live beyond myself. I like to think that this book and the opportunity to walk other cancer patients through *their* ordeals are among the reasons why I am still here while Bruce is not. Ultimately, the answer to the question "Why me?" in this context remains for you to script.

Indeed, life after cancer is not about the residual stress from having had it or the strange guilt of having survived it.

If you have gone through cancer or are dealing with it now, you have seen life on the edge. You have stared death in the face. No one can—or should—go through that experience and come out the other side as the same person. While you may be relieved to reclaim some normalcy in your life when your cancer treatments are over, "getting back to normal" is neither the goal nor a laudable result. Your life post-cancer should be *other* than normal. It should be *better* than normal. If you are asking yourself why you survived or what you did to deserve the second chance you have been given, the answer lies in the improvements you make post-cancer.

Some months into my treatment and remission, a good friend and colleague told me that the extreme emotions involved in having cancer and going through treatment would pass. He had endured his own wife's breast cancer treatment shortly before I was diagnosed with leukemia. I remember saying to him at the time that I hoped on some level that those emotions, those feelings associated with having and being treated for cancer, would remain. Of course, I was not talking about the fear and uncertainty. I was talking about the sheer joy of being alive and reveling in what life had to offer.

Like a lot of cancer patients, I developed a keen sense for these things during my experience. I experienced—and continue to experience—unbridled joy at being able to go outside and feel the air on my face—something that was denied to me during my initial treatment. I often express how all of the rest of my life post-cancer is "bonus time." I never take it for granted. I have come to the realization that, as Henry David Thoreau wrote, "Heaven is under our feet as well as over our heads."[134]

Others noticed the changes in me as well. Almost immediately upon my return to work, I started spending extensive

---

time in Alabama in connection with a large toxic tort/environmental case my firm was handling. After an enormous, years-long litigation, it came to a very successful conclusion for our clients. When I returned to our New York office, the senior partner of the firm told me that he had noticed a marked improvement in my work and how I handled my aspects of the case, and he asked me what had triggered that sea change in my performance. "I had cancer," I told him simply. As I explained to him, as a result of going through and winning my battle against cancer, I was different. My former timidity in the professional realm was gone. I feared things less. I was less wary of speaking my mind and asserting myself. Cancer had made me a better lawyer and, I hope, a more improved person.

Earlier in my life, my ego often had gotten the best (or perhaps the *worst*) of me. I was athletic. I was popular. I was cocky. Too often I could be sarcastic and, although I was never intentionally mean, I was not always sensitive to how other people felt or how what I said might affect them. I would make jokes at other people's expense, meeting any pushback or hurt feelings with "I was just kidding" (which I was, not that it mattered to my targets).

Then cancer, and all that it entailed, happened. Although it was mostly unconscious, with moments of directed lucidity, I changed. Cancer had changed *me*. The cockiness of supposed invincibility and self-assuredness was gone. Any sense of superiority I must have had went with it. I was more generous and more giving. Instead of merely being *nice*, I had discovered how to be *kind*—perhaps by virtue of the many kindnesses bestowed upon *me*.

All of this came home to me one day when a good friend whom I had met before my cancer told me that he had described me to his father-in-law not only as someone who "beat the hell out of cancer," but someone who was "the nicest, most generous person" he knew. I doubt whether he could honestly have described me in those terms pre-cancer. And while I have come to realize that being a "better" person is a road, not a destination, his words let me know that at least I was on the right path.

Your goal as a cancer survivor as well should be not only to *feel* better but to *be* better. As pastor Charles Swindoll advised, life is ten percent what happens to you and ninety percent how you react to it.[135] Be a better person, friend, spouse, father or child. Whereas many who suffer from cancer do not get a second chance to enjoy all that life has to offer, *you have been given that chance.* If for no other reason than the simple fact that you owe it to those people who were not given a second chance, as well as your loved ones who have helped you through your cancer and, most important, yourself, you should strive to be better in any way you can. Avoid arguments. Let insults or slights slide off your back. Be more patient and more courteous with people. Take the time to appreciate. Thank people who do things for you, even (and particularly) if those things are everyday chores. Tell the people you love that you love them instead of waiting until the time is "right." After all, isn't it *always* the right time for that? Realize that, as I have told many people who have pointed out certain "problems" in life, if you and the people you love are healthy, everything else in life—be it money, work or daily hassles—is a cakewalk.

Further, be *inspiring*. Nothing will set the stage for others more than how we *act*. Be a good example. There is a scene toward the end of the movie *Saving Private Ryan* where Tom Hanks's character, mortally wounded, tells Matt Damon's character to "earn" the sacrifices made on his behalf. Show those around you that *you* have earned the second chance you have received by being a better person. Treat life with

---

135 C. Swindoll, *Strengthening Your Grip.*

the sanctity and reverence that it deserves. Do not betray the loyalty, friendship and support given to you during your ordeal by returning to your status quo ante, replete with unhealthy habits, after you have defeated your cancer. Many of the nutritional suggestions in this book and elsewhere are appropriate not only while you are sick or in treatment but for the rest of your life. Avoid unhealthy foods that do your body little, if any, good (and may do it substantial damage).

If you avoided exercise before you got sick, resolve to stick with an exercise routine to keep your immune system pumped up. If, like me, you were someone who worked constantly, well into the wee hours of the night, get more rest so your body can rejuvenate. And work meditation of some sort into your routine as well, even if it consists only of sitting in a quiet environment and breathing deeply. You will be amazed by how closing yourself off even for a few minutes to reflect can improve your life.

Moreover, strive to take your changed perspectives beyond your immediate world and family. Your experiences can and should live beyond yourself. Give some of your time to a worthy cause. Volunteer at your local church, synagogue or mosque. Serve on the board of your children's school. Give a few hours a week to charity (and involve your other family members in your activities).

If you don't have the time or interpersonal skills to work with a charitable organization, there are many other ways that you can use your ordeal to help others. Unfortunately, people are being diagnosed with cancer every day, including whichever cancer you had. Let the hospital where you were treated or your doctor know that you are available for other cancer patients who may need the perspective and encouragement you have gained by your experiences.

During and after my treatment, I occasionally visited the hospital ward where I was treated and asked if any of the patients wanted to speak with me. I have readily offered my phone number and time to others who have been diagnosed with cancer. Helping them express themselves and giving them encouragement that, like me, they could beat their cancer, helped me as much as it hopefully helped them. You are now a veteran of the cancer wars, and your words—and the example you set—may be what transforms another person from a cancer victim into a cancer survivor. What greater gift is there to give than that?

Celebrate. As Albert Einstein once said: "*There are two ways to live: You can live as if nothing is a miracle; you can live as if everything is a miracle.*" Once you have survived your cancer, Einstein's second option should inform your approach to life. Celebrate everything that is worth celebrating. When someone says to me, often without even thinking about it, "Have a nice day," I often respond that "Every day is a nice day," because, if you and the people you love are healthy, every day *is* a nice day.

Regardless of how old you are, celebrate your birthday. My friends, making note of the gray creeping into my hair and the white in my beard when I let it grow, sometimes ask me if I mind getting older. I always answer them, "Compared to what?" Indeed, now that you have survived your cancer, you have *new* birthdays, including the day you were diagnosed and the day you went into remission. Celebrate those days as well. They are the anniversaries of your rebirth and your entry into a new life.

APPENDIX A

WHAT TO BRING TO THE HOSPITAL

The following is a suggested list of items you may want to bring with you if you are going to be spending extended time in the hospital. You will need to clear any items on the list that the hospital may not want you bringing from home (e.g., your own blankets or pillows) or items that may not be advisable during your treatment (certain toiletries, eye drops, etc.).

Comfortable clothes for daytime use
Slip-on shoes
Pajamas or doctor's scrubs
Slippers
Warm socks
Sweater or sweatshirt
Absorbent robe
Toiletries (note that you may not be able to tolerate certain usual toiletries, including colognes/perfumes, deodorant and toothpastes)
Biotene toothpaste
Flushable baby wipes
Lubricant eye drops
Inspirational reading material
Stationery and pens
Calming music

Aromatherapy oils
Family pictures
Head covering
Blanket
Pillow
Communication/entertainment devices with headphones
(cell phones, laptops, DVD player, iPad, MP3 player)
Comedy DVDs or recordings
Sugar-free sucking candies or lollypops

APPENDIX B

WHAT TO BRING TO OUTPATIENT TREATMENTS

The following is a suggested list of items you may want to bring with you when you go for outpatient treatments, if those treatments will take longer than several minutes to administer. As with the items listed in Appendix A, you should clear any items on the list that may not be advisable during your treatment (certain toiletries, eye drops, etc.) or may be disruptive to other patients receiving treatment at the same time as you.

Slip-on shoes
Slippers
Warm socks
Sweater or sweatshirt
Inspirational reading material
Calming music
Aromatherapy oils
Head covering
Lap blanket or throw
Support pillow for your head or back
Communication/entertainment devices with headphones (cell phones, laptops, DVD player, iPad, MP3 player)
Comedy DVDs or recordings
Work
Bottled water

Sugar-free sucking candies or lollypops
Treatment buddy (a friend or relative who can accompany
you to treatments)

APPENDIX C

PREPARATIONS LIST

The following is a list of information you may want to assemble and issues that you may want to address and make sure someone is taking care of while you are hospitalized or going through your treatment.

- Bill payments: Make sure that any bills that may have to be paid during your treatment are either being paid through an automatic payment program or that whoever will be paying them has the account information, payment amounts and addresses to send payments.
- Bank account information and contact numbers: If anyone is handling your financial affairs, including deposits to your accounts or bill payments, while you are undergoing treatment, he should have your bank account numbers and contact numbers for individuals at your bank with whom you work.
- Investment information and contact numbers: Same as above—whoever is handling your financial affairs should have the names, addresses, contact numbers and account numbers for your investments.
- Medical insurance policy information and contact numbers.
- Will: A copy of your will should be left with your attorney or personal representative (which may include your spouse or anyone else you designate as the executor of your estate under the terms of your will).

- Power of attorney (which should be given to whoever is granted the power of attorney so that he can exercise the authority on your behalf).
- Shopping: Make sure arrangements are made to have someone (preferably someone other than your immediate family members or caretakers) take care of basic shopping needs, such as groceries or items you may need during your convalescence. This list will vary for each person, but some of the basics that should be covered include: (i) food shopping, including a list of any food items that should not be purchased for you (for example, because you cannot tolerate them or have chosen not to eat them during your treatment, or because someone in your home is allergic or sensitive to such foods); (ii) medicines for you or others in your family; (iii) school or work supplies; (iv) household items (including cleaning products, paper goods, etc.); and (v) pet supplies (especially if someone else is caring for your pets during your treatment).
- Meal preparation: Make sure people are willing and available to prepare meals for you if you are unable to do so for yourself, and advise those people as to what you can and cannot eat. You should reach out to at least a half-dozen friends who are willing to help out, and ask one of them to organize meal preparations with the others.
- Babysitting.
- Children's schedules (getting to and from school, extracurricular activities, carpools).
- Funeral arrangements.
- Life insurance policy information and contact numbers: As with bank and investment accounts, the person who is handling your financial affairs should have the name, address and contact numbers for your life insurance policies, the account numbers for those policies and the amount of coverage of each policy.

BIBLIOGRAPHY

Books

American Cancer Society, Complete Guide to Complementary & Alternative Cancer Therapies (2d ed. 2009)

Beliveau, Richard and Gingras, Denis, *Foods that Fight Cancer*, New York: Random House, 2006.

Buckman, Robert, "Providing Emotional Support," in Yount, Lisa, *Cancer: Contemporary Issues Companion*, Farmington Hills, MI: Greenhaven Press, 2000.

Campbell, T. C. and Campbell, T. M., *The China Study*, Dallas, TX, Benbella Books, 2006.

Chapters of the Fathers 1:14; 2:21

Congreve, William, *The Mourning Bride* I, Oxford University Press 1928

Gorter, Robert and Peper, Erik, *Fighting Cancer: A Nontoxic Approach to Treatment*, Berkeley, CA: North Atlantic Books, 2011.

Groddeck, Georg, *The Book of the It* (1923).

Keane, M. and Chace, D., *What to Eat If You Have Cancer: Healing Foods that Boost Your Immune System*, updated Second Ed. New York: McGraw-Hill, 2007.

Schorr, Andrew and Thomas, Mary, *The Web-Savvy Patient: An Insider's Guide to Navigating the Internet When Facing Medical Crisis* (2011).

Servan-Schreiber, David, *Anticancer: A New Way of Life*, New York: Viking, 2008.

United States Department of Agriculture, *Dietary Guidelines for Americans*, 2010

Wein, Rabbi Berel, *Buy Green Bananas*, Brooklyn, N.Y. Shaar Press, 1999.

Articles

N. B. Alitheen, et al., "Cytotoxic Effects of Commercial Wheatgrass and Fiber Towards Human Acute Promyelocytic Leukemia Cells (HL60)," *Pak J Pharm Sci.* (July 2011): 24(3):243–50.

American Cancer Society, "Patient's Bill of Rights: What is the Patient's Bill of Rights," http://www.cancer.org/Treatment/FindingandPayingforTreatment/UnderstandingFinancialandLegalMatters/patients-bill-of-rights.

American Cancer Society's review of metabolic treatments, http://www.cancer.org/Treatment/TreatmentsandSideEffects/ComplementaryandAlternativeMedicine/DietandNutrition/metabolic-therapy.

American Cancer Society, "Spirituality and Prayer," http://www.cancer.org/Treatment/TreatmentsandSideEffects/ComplementaryandAlternativeMedicine/MindBodyandSpirit/spirituality-and-prayer.

M. Barrera, "The Effects of Interactive Music Therapy on Hospitalized Children with Cancer: a Pilot Study," *Psycho-Oncology*, vol. 11, no. 5 (September/October 2002): 378–388.

S. Barrett, "Questionable Cancer Therapies," http://www.quackwatch.com/01QuackeryRelatedTopics/cancer.html.

G. Bar-Sela, et al., Wheat Grass Juice May Improve Hematological Toxicity Related to Chemotherapy in Breast Cancer Patients: A Pilot Study," *Nutrition and Cancer*, vol. 58, no. 1 (2007), 43–48.

T. Brasky, et al., "Serum Phospholipid Fatty Acids and Prostate Cancer Risk: Results from the Prostate Cancer Prevention Trial," *Am J. Epidemiol.* (2011): 173(12): 1429–1439.

T. Brasky, et al., "Plasma Phospholipid Fatty Acids and Prostate Cancer Risk in the SELECT Trial," *JNCI J.* Natl Cancer Inst (2013): 10.1093/jnci/djt174.

E. H. Byun, et al., "TLR4 Signaling Inhibitory Pathway Induced by Green Tea Polyphenol Epigallocatechin-3-Gallate through 67-kDa Laminin Receptor," *J. Immun.* 185, no. 1 (July 2010): 33–45.

B. Cassileth, PhD, and A. Vickers, PhD, "Massage Therapy for Symptom Control: Outcome Study at a Major Cancer Center," *Journal of Pain and Symptom Management*, vol. 28, no. 3 (September 2004): 244–249.

A. Chatham, MPhil, MTh, MSW, "Our Emotions Can Create White Blood Cells," *Healing Our World*, vol. 31, no. 4 (2011), Hippocrates Health Institute 2011.

G. H. Christ and A. Christ, "Current Approaches to Helping Children Cope with a Parent's Terminal Illness," *CA: Cancer Guide for Clinicians*, vol. 56, no. 4 (July/August 2006): 197–212.

A. S. Daba and O. U. Ezeronye, "Anti-Cancer Effects of Polysaccharides Isolated From Higher Basidiomycetes Mushrooms," *African Journal of Biotechnology*, vol. 2(12) (December 2003): 672–678.

G. DeNardo and S. DeNardo, "Turning the Heat on Cancer," *Cancer Biotherapy and Radiopharmaceuticals*, vol. 23, no. 6 (2008): 671–680.

"Does Sugar Feed Cancer," http://www.sciencedaily.com/releases/2009/08/090817184539.htm.

R. I. M. Dunbar, et al., "Social Laughter is Correlated with an Elevated Pain Threshold," *Proc. R. Soc. B* (August 2011): 5.

J. Dwyer, et al., "The Effect of Religious Concentration and Affiliation on County Cancer Mortality Rates," *Journal of Health and Social Behavior* 31(2) (1990): 185–202.

D. Eilam, et al., "Threat Detection: Behavioral Practices in Animals and Humans," *Neurosci Biobehav Rev.* (March 2011): 35(4):999–1006.

F. I. Fawzy, et al., "Effects of an Early Structured Psychiatric Intervention, Coping and Affective State on Recurrence and Survival 6 Years Later," *Arch Gen Psychiatry* (1993): 50:681–689.

F. I. Fawzy, et al., "Malignant Melanoma: Effects of a Brief, Structured Psychiatric Intervention on Survival and Recurrence at 10-Year Follow-Up," *Arch Gen Psychiatry* (2003): 60:100–103.

D. Fellowes, et al., "Aromatherapy and Massage for Symptom Relief in Patients with Cancer," *Cochrane Database of Systematic Reviews 2008*, no. 4. Art. No.: CD002287; doi:10.1002/14651858.CD002287.pub3.

E. Filipski, et al., "Disruption of Circadian Coordination and Malignant Growth," *Cancer Causes Control* (May 2006: 17(4):509–514.

J. Finley, et al., "Cancer-Protective Properties of High Selenium Broccoli," *J. Agric. Food Chem.* (2001): 49: 2679–2683.

G. Gellert, et al., "Survival of Breast Cancer Patients Receiving Adjunctive Psychosocial Support Therapy: A 10-Year Follow-Up Study," *Journal of Clinical Oncology* (1993): 11:66–69.

S. Gould, "The Median Isn't the Message," http://cancerguide.org/median_not_msg.html;

E. S. Harris, "Adolescent Bereavement Following the Death of a Parent: An Exploratory Study," *Child Psychiatry Hum. Dev.* (Summer 1991): 21(4):267–281.

"Helping Children when a Family Member has Cancer: When a Child has Lost a Parent," http://www.cancer.org/Treatment/ChildrenandCancer/HelpingChildrenWhenaFamilyMemberHasCancer/WhenaChildHasLostaParent/index.

S. M. Hennings, "Bioavailability and Antioxidant Activity of Tea Flavanols After Consumption of Green Tea, Black Tea and Green Tea Extract Supplement," *Amer. Journal of Clinical Nutrition* (2004): 80(6):1558–1564.

B. Hildebrandt, et al., "The Cellular and Molecular Basis for Hyperthermia," *Crit Rev Oncol/Hematol* (July 2002): 43(1):33–56.

R. Hilliard, "Music Therapy in Hospice and Palliative Care: A Review of the Empirical Data," *Evid. Based Complement. Alternat. Med.* (June 2005): 2(2):173–178.

A. Hoicowitz, et al., "How Color Affects Mood," http://jr-science.wcp.muohio.edu/nsfall99/labpacketArticles/Final1.HowColorAffectsMoo.html;

R. Jahnke, et al., "A Comprehensive Review of Health Benefits of Qigong and Tai Chi," *Am J Health Promot.* (July/August 2010): 24(6): e1–e25.

B. Kaada and O. Torsteinbo, "Increase of Plasma B-Endorphins in Connective Tissue Massage," *General Pharmacology: The Vascular System*, vol. 20, no. 4 (1989): 487–489.

I. S. Lee and G. J. Lee, "Effects of Lavender Aromatherapy on Insomnia and Depression in Women College Students," *Taehan Kanho Hakhoe Chi.* (Feb 2006): 36(1):136–143.

M. Leitzmann, et al., "Dietary Intake of n-3 and n-6 Fatty Acids and the Risk of Prostate Cancer," *Am J. Clin Nutr* (2004): 80: 204–216.

Y. Li, et al., "Sulforathane, a Dietary Component of Broccoli/Broccoli Sprouts, Inhibits Breast Cancer Stem Cells," *Clin Cancer Res.* (May 1, 2010): 16(9): 2580–2590.

N. Motomura, et al., "Reduction of Mental Stress with Lavender Odorant," *Percept Mot Skills.* (December 2001): 93(3): 713–718.

M. Myzak and R. Dashwood, "Chemoprevention by Sulforathane: Keep One Eye Beyond Keap1," *Cancer Lett.* (February 28, 2006): 233(2): 208–218.

National Institute of Health's Dietary Supplement Fact Sheet for Valerian, http://ods.od.nih.gov/factsheets/valerian.

D. Ornish, et al., "Intensive Lifestyle Changes May Affect the Progression of Prostate Cancer," *Journal of Urology*, vol. 174, no. 3 (September 2005): 1065–1070.

J. Post-White, et al., "Therapeutic Massage and Healing Touch Improve Symptoms in Cancer," *Integrative Cancer Therapies* (2003): 2(4): 332–344.

S. Reuter, et al., "Oxidative Stress, Inflammation and Cancer: How are they Linked?" *Free Radoc Biol. Med.* (December 2010): 49(11): 1603–1616.

D. P. Rose, et al., "Diet and Breast Cancer," American Institute for Cancer Research, Plenum Press (1994): 83-91.

A. Sadeh, "Stress, Trauma and Sleep in Children," Child and Adolescent Psychiatric Clinics of North America, (1996): 5(3):685–700.

M. Sartippour, et al., "The Combination of Green Tea and Tamoxifen is Effective Against Breast Cancer," *Carcinogenesis* (2006): 27(12): 2424–2433.

J. Satin, et al., "Depression as a Predictor of Disease Progression and Mortality in Cancer Patients: A Meta-Analysis," *Cancer*, vol. 115, no. 22 (November 15, 2009): 5349–5361.

S. Sephton and D. Spiegel, "Circadian Disruption in Cancer: A Neuroendocrine-Immune Pathway from Stress to Disease?" *Brain, Behavior and Immunity*, vol. 17 (2003): 321–328.

Y. Shao, et al., "Enhancement of the Antineoplastic Effect of Mitomycin C by Dietary Fat," *Cancer Res.* (1994): 54: 6452–6457.

Y. Shao, et al., "Dietary Menhaden Oil Enhances Mitomycin C Antitumor Activity Toward Human Mammary Carcinoma MX-1," *Lipids* (1995): 30: 1035–1045.

R. B. Shekelle, et al., "Psychological Depression and 17-Year Risk of Death from Cancer," *Psychosom Med.* (1981): 43: 117–125.

R. Skopec, "Mechanism Linking Aggression Stress through Inflammation to Cancer," *J. Cancer Sci Ther* (2011): 3:6: 134–139.

D. Spiegel, et al., "Effect of Psychosocial Treatment on Survival of Patients with Metastatic Breast Cancer," *Lancet* (1989) 2: 888–891.

"Sugar and Cancer: Is There a Connection," http://www.caring4cancer.com/go/cancer/nutrition/questions/sugar-and-cancer-is-there-a-connection.htm.

"Tea and Cancer Prevention: Strengths and Limits of the Evidence," http://www.cancer.gov/cancertopics/factsheet/prevention/tea.

R. Ulrich, "Effects of Healthcare Environmental Design on Medical Outcomes," *IADH* International Academy for Design and Health (2001), 53.

US Department of Agriculture "Dietary Guidelines for Americans," (2010).

U.S. News & World Report comprehensive ranking of hospitals nationwide, http://health.usnews.com/best-hospitals.

J. van de Zee, "Heating the Patient: A Promising Approach?" *Ann Oncol.* (August 2002) 13(8): 1173–1184.

W. C. Wang, et al., "The Effects of Tai Chi on Psychosocial Well-Being: A Systematic Review of Randomized Controlled Trials," J Acupunct Meridian Stud. (September 2009): 2(3): 171–181.

P. Wust, et al., "Hyperthermia in Combined Treatment of Cancer," *Lancet Oncol.* (August 2002): 3(8): 487–497.

Young-Joon Surh, "Cancer Chemoprevention with Dietary Phytochemicals," *Nature*, vol. 3 (October 2003): 768–780.

INDEX

ABOUT THE AUTHOR

Howard Bressler has been married to his wife, Ceci, for twenty-two years. They have two daughters and live on Long Island, New York. Howard has been practicing law in New York City for more than twenty years, with a heavy emphasis on toxic tort (chemical exposure), product liability and environmental actions. He has worked on cases, including some of the largest toxic tort litigations in the country, in various jurisdictions in the United States. Throughout his career, Howard has both defended against and prosecuted the claims of people who claimed to have suffered injuries, including various types of cancer, from exposure to toxic substances. Part of his work over the years has involved researching and reviewing scientific studies and working with experts to understand whether and how various substances and stimuli cause illness, and how to best explain those issues to judges and juries.

When he was diagnosed with Acute Promyelocytic Leukemia (APL) in August 2000, during his subsequent treatments, through his bouts with Stevens-Johnson Syndrome and in the course of researching and writing this book, Howard tapped into much of what he has learned from his experiences in terms of reviewing, vetting and applying scientific studies to understand the initiation, progression and treatment of disease, and explaining these issues in layman's terms. In this book, he also has applied his legal skills in evaluating and setting forth issues relating to patients' and workplace rights, as well as estate planning and other practical issues cancer patients face. Howard himself underwent extensive treatment for his leukemia, including high-dose chemotherapy and a then-experimental course of treatment with arsenic trioxide (which has since been incorporated into the regular regimen for APL patients). He has also counseled several other cancer patients in their battles against the disease.